HAND IN HAND WITH ANGELS

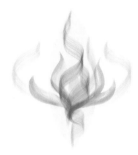

To David
I hope you make many angel friends
in these pages
love from Kathleen

Kathleen Pepper

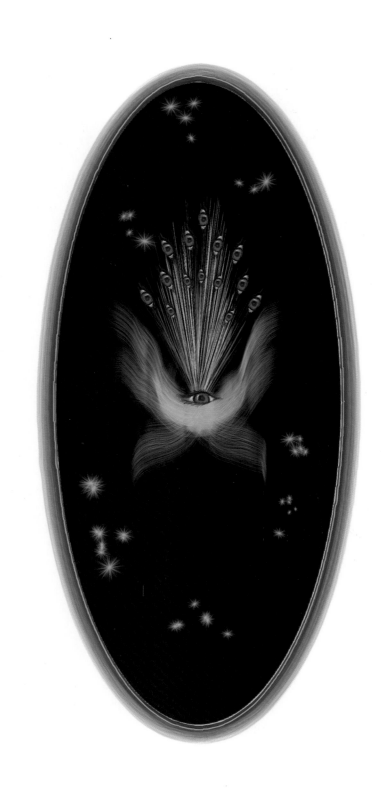

Hand in Hand with Angels

Kathleen Pepper

POLAIR PUBLISHING

LONDON

www.polairpublishing.co.uk

First published October 2010

British Library Cataloguing-in-Publication Data
A catalogue record for this book is available
from the British Library
ISBN 978-1-905398-21-8

DISCLAIMER
*Meditation and complementary therapies are
no substitute for medical advice when needed.*

TO ROY

ACKNOWLEDGMENTS

First of all I must thank my husband, Roy, my computer 'angel', without whom
this book would still be in my imagination. He rescues me from all the things
that happen when I am at a computer. Secondly, thank you to Colum Hayward
for his helpful support, patience, editing and advice; to Morgan Hesmondhalgh
for her illustrations of angels; to Lesley, for her encouragement throughout the
writing of the book; my friends Meher and Sharry for all their help, especially
at tough times; to Jo, Ron, Geraldine, Drica, all in my KEYS meditation group
and yoga groups for their suggestions and feedback over the years; and to all
who have attended my angel workshops since 1998 and have been the first to
try the angels' ideas. Thank you to Judy Levy of Geo Art, for the crystal angel
photographed on page 42, to the White Eagle Publishing Trust, for permission
to use a number of extracts from White Eagle's teaching, and to Paneurhythmy
Circle of Joy for the Peter Deunov prayer on p. 39. Thank you to Theolyn
Cortens, Jacqui Malone and Jenny Dent for their reading and reviews. If
I have forgotten anyone, I apologize. You know who you
are and I thank you very much.

*Set in Minion, Helvetica and Sassafras at the publisher
and printed in the Hashemite Republic of Jordan
at National Press, Amman*

CONTENTS

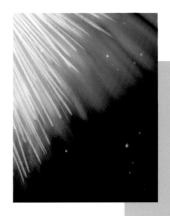

PROLOGUE

'Write about us', said the angels.

'What shall I write?' I asked.

'Write our messages.
Our messages need to go out into the world.
We need to wake people up to our presence.
We need to wake people up to all the possibilities of our
partnership and friendship with people.
Write that we are always here.
Wherever you go in your daily life, we are with you.
When you are in your car, or travelling by bus, train or
plane, we are with you.
When you sit by the river, admiring the ripples on the
water and the reflections on its surface, we are with you.
When you lie on the soft green grass in the park,
the meadow, your garden, we are with you in
every blade of grass.
When you think things are getting tough,
we are with you.
When you are happy, when you are joyful,
when you are loving, we are with you.
We are with you at your birth into your world
And at your passing into the World of Light,
We are always there, we are always with you.

'How will the partnership between angels and people
develop?', I asked.

'Write about us, talk about us, spread the word and
our message will spread far and wide. Be fearless, as we
know you are. Even your friend who thought we were
"creepy" now believes, is beginning to use affirmations,
to buy angel gifts, to wear angel pins.

'Remember us.

'Remember we are always with you.
When you sleep, you come to us in our
world (and your true world!)
When you awaken, you forget.
We honour you for the way you continue in faith,
Clinging to the dim memories of your dreams,
Obeying the guidance of your soul,
Walking, often blindly, through your life,
But always walking your path,
Walking your talk.

'And one day, you will
RE-MEMBER!
And all will slip back into its rightful place.
You will know that people and angels work together,
Are part of the same family,
The same team.
So know that we are always there with you.
Remember us, for we remember you.'

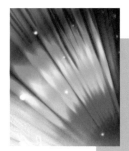

Angel Message

(A message from the Angel of Vision, received especially for this book in July 2009)

CREATE!

Every day, create and recreate
The beauty of the earth!
Create love in your hearts, O people of Gaia.
Our angel work is to create and maintain form
And then with your help to bring it into physical manifestation.
This vision we share with you.
Ours is the vision
Yours are the physical hands
That perform the task.
Ask us and we are with you
Sharing our vision
And giving you inspiration,
Providing strength, courage and ability
For all your needs,
To heal the environment.
You are of Earth and in your physical beauty you are indeed Earth.
We are the bridge from spirit to matter:
You are the bridge from matter to spirit!
You live in two worlds and we are your partners.

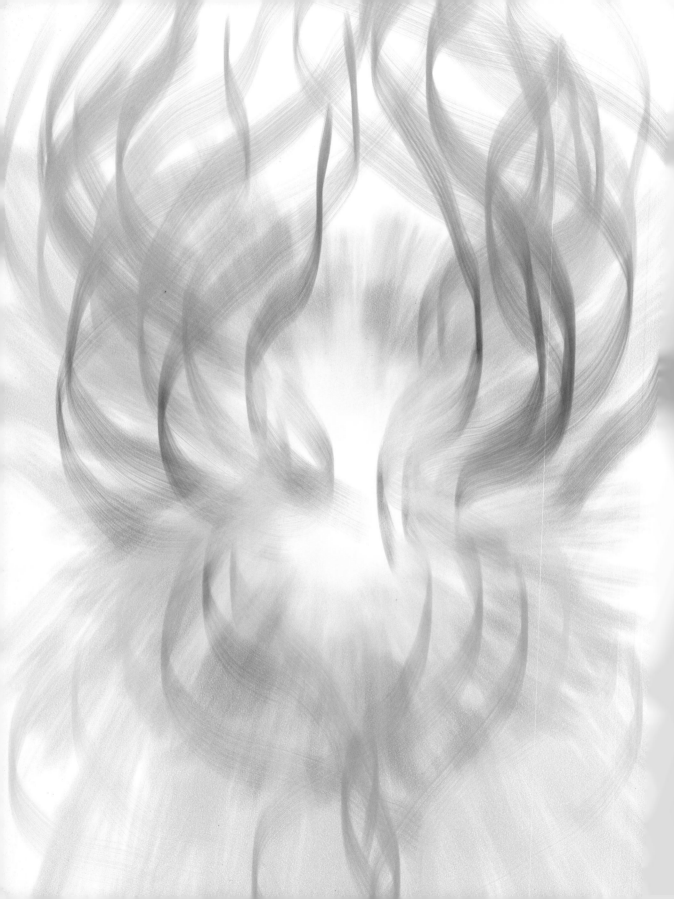

1.

Introducing Angels

Life is full of mystery. It is like a tangled ball of coloured wool that we need to unravel one bit at a time. The ball is full of colour but nothing can be done with it. Life is like that. When we undo one knot at a time, we begin to create a wonderful tapestry of colour and vibrancy. Angels are everywhere and will help us to untangle life's great mysteries.

ANGELS are coming back into our lives. Of course, they never really went away. They are all around us. They have always been there, speaking to us in our dreams, our inner voice, intuition, and our conscience. But sometime during the last two or three hundred years, after the Industrial Revolution, people became more rational and intellectual. They reduced their use of the right brain, the intuitive and creative side, and began to trust the left brain, which is the logical and intellectual side. Children began school at age four or five and learned to read, write and calculate and to think rationally in order to know how to play their part in the world: to drive the bus, as it were. The creative and intuitive aspect of their lives took more of a back seat. Only some of us, the ones who were always told off for daydreaming, had a rich inner life. People became more reluctant to talk of their inner experiences, including their meetings with angels and spirit guides, afraid of being laughed at.

In some ways, the age we live in has become rather sceptical and cynical because we think that if we can't see something, touch it or feel it, then it isn't there. We do know, however, that there are things that can only be seen with a microscope or telescope, or with electronic and even electromagnetic scans, so we know plenty of things that cannot be seen with the naked eye. People have grown to mistrust their inner vision, and to dismiss it as 'pure imagination'.

What a wonderful concept, 'pure imagination'! The secret of communicating with and seeing angels is to do it through the heart and to trust your imagination and intuition. Angels do not want us to worship them, because worship is for God alone. They only ask that we love them and work selflessly with them for the highest good of all. Angels are a part of life's mystery. Try too hard and the mystery cannot be unravelled; an angel's wing is only glimpsed and then disappears.

There are traditions about angels that are thousands of years old and some of the most magnificent art has been produced about angels. Go into any cathedral or art gallery to see the results of someone's artistic vision of angels in stained glass, statues or paintings. The results of inner vision are then plain to view. The artists have worked with their inner vision to produce angel artefacts that are easily spotted in our material world.

Cathy and her husband were staying in a hotel in an Indian town when he had a bad fall. It was the last day before travelling to the airport to return home. He had bruised ribs and was also running a high temperature, so there was fear of malaria. A general strike was threatened. How would they get to the airport? Also, there was no time to try to get medical attention. These fears went through Cathy's mind, leaving her in a state of panic. The hotel room was on the fourth or fifth floor. It was opposite tree tops, where the only birds to be seen were vultures and birds of prey. She asked the angels for a sign that they were near, giving their support. Not long after, a tiny black and white bird landed on the balcony outside. It was the only small bird they had seen. It was there for quite some time. Cathy felt very supported, and she and her husband returned safely home, where he was able to receive medical attention.

So what are angels? They are Beings of Light, who work with the Source of All-That-Is (that is, God, or All Light, or whatever your favourite term is for the Creator) and who are dedicated totally to the light. God works through the angels and they exist to do His–Her will. Angels are all around us. They are everywhere. Whatever we do, wherever we go, our angel friends are with us. We live on a planet of freewill, so unless we are in serious danger, angels will wait until asked before they help. Spiritual law is that we have to ask for angel help when we need it. If the request is for the highest good of all concerned, that help is there. The angels will always help, though we do not always get what we expect! But be assured that a team of angels of light surround us with support and will give a sign of their presence if asked for it.

Looking at the story opposite, maybe it is not surprising that it was a bird that meant so much to Cathy in her crisis. There is a long tradition that angels disguise themselves as birds.* The teacher White Eagle has this to say about birds:

> 'The birds bring happiness, they release the soul to spiritual realms. You must needs be happy when you hear the song of birds; listening to music or the song of birds, a chord awakens in you which carries you into the spiritual worlds. Do not listen with the mind alone, although you need an intelligent mind to comprehend music; but the chords of the heart should be struck and then you are released— you fly; you overcome earthiness, like birds you are able to fly, released to the spiritual worlds, and your heart records happiness.'

Angels and angel-like beings are to be found all over the world and in many different traditions. The first known references to them are to be found in the oldest traditions we have—the Babylonian, Zoroastrian, Assyrian and Chaldean. The Indian traditions do not mention angels as such. The nearest term is *deva*, which means Shining One.

*See *The Return of the Bird Tribes*, by Ken Carey

Buddhists refer to *dakini*, a goddess figure or enlightened female energy. Both Hindus and Buddhists talk in terms of gods and goddesses, rather than angels. The middle-eastern and western monotheistic theologies prevent belief in other divinities, but angels are part of their tradition. *Deva* is a term often used now to refer to an angelic being that works with the nature kingdom, like plants or crystals.

The best-known definition of angels puts them into what are known as 'choirs' to show all the orders of angels. An early Christian writer who is now known as Pseudo-Dionysius devized this system in the fifth or sixth century.* In his system, there are nine orders of angelic beings, the first order or sphere being the highest.

There have been many attempts to classify angels and archangels and it can be very confusing. It's as if the angels themselves like to keep us guessing and imply that it is only human beings who have to have categories and classifications. Perhaps the only way the human brain can understand things is to attempt to define them.

For simplicity, though, I will follow the system of Pseudo-Dionysius. The first sphere consists of angels who serve as heavenly counsellors and are the seraphim, cherubim and thrones. **The Seraphim** are the highest order of the spiritual hierarchy. Their name means 'firemakers', 'carriers of warmth' or 'ardour'. They are the keepers of divine love. This love consumes them and keeps them close to the throne of God. These celestial beings are thought to surround the throne of God and to sing the music of the spheres and regulate the movement of the heavens. The universe is stated to have been brought into being through sound and the sacred sound of creation is thought to be the mantra 'OM' or 'AUM', so it is easy to accept that sound and harmony create and maintain the universe.

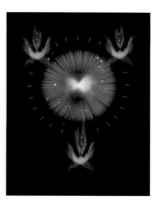

Call on Uriel when you want to work with the seraphim. His name means 'Fire of God' and he holds the energies of love and truth. He is also an angel of transformation. The seraphim

*Encyclopedia of Angels, by Rosemary Ellen Guiley

will help us to work with charity, goodwill, compassion, unconditional love and comfort and help us to release and heal selfishness, hatred, dislike, distrust, abuse and evil.

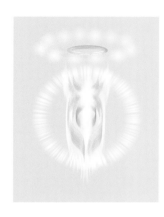

The Cherubim, who form the next tier of angels, are guardians of light and the stars. The name is from the Hebrew word *kerub*, meaning either 'fullness of knowledge' or 'one who intercedes'. They are the voice of divine wisdom and have a deep insight into divine secrets. Though they are far away from humanity, they filter the divine light throughout the universe to touch our lives. (They are not the same as the cherubs who look like naked babies and decorate greetings cards!) In the Koran, it is said that the tears that Archangel Michael weeps over the wrongdoing of the faithful forms the cherubim. They are said to have six wings and are full of all-seeing eyes. They constantly sing praises to God.

Cherubiel, whose name comes from cherubim, oversees this order of angels. They will assist us to expand our ability to work with knowledge, spiritual wisdom, truth, enlightenment, discernment and revelation. They will help us to work on releasing falsehood, deception, illusion and ignorance.

The Thrones are the companion angels of the planets, such as Mercury, Venus and Mars. Gaia, the planetary spirit or Angel of Earth, is a throne and the guardian of our world. We can work in harmony with Gaia by being responsible towards the planet and the environment, by living as simple a life as possible, or by regular prayer, such as the White Eagle Lodge advises.* At a more functional level, we can recycle things we don't want by donating through charity shops, or to local fundraising events. If you have a garden, and even in many cities now, you can recycle your kitchen waste into compost. You can make a corner of your garden into a peaceful area for meditation. You can build up a good relationship with the thrones by working with the one who is special to our own planet.

Raziel is the contact archangel for the thrones. He is

*As I write, the latest White Eagle book is called EARTH HEALER, and has some very helpful angel prayers and attunements in it.

thought to guard the secrets of the universe and is keeper of the Book of Raziel. His name means 'secret of God' or 'Angel of Mysteries'. The Book of Raziel is said to have been the first book ever written in Heaven and to be made of sapphire and contain the secrets of the cosmos. Raziel teaches that the most profound knowledge is not found through reading books but from the heart. Thrones will help us to understand and live a life of equality, fairness, divine justice, selflessness, open-mindedness, creativity and inspiration. We can work with them to release prejudice, narrow-mindedness, rash outbursts, and inconsiderateness.

The second sphere of angels is those who work as heavenly governors. They are the dominions, virtues and powers. **The Dominions** are like managers and organizers, and they arrange the activities of angelic groups who are lower in rank than they are. They are obedient to the Source of All-That-Is and their work is connected to our earthly reality, but like government officials or managing directors, they do not necessarily know individuals for they manage and organize those who do. You can think of them as divine bureaucrats. They also integrate the spiritual and physical worlds. They know the divine plan and maintain the sacred order of the universe. Call on Zadkiel when you need to work with dominions. Archangel Zadkiel, whose name means 'righteousness of God', is one of the seven archangels who stand before the throne and presence of God. Ask for help from dominions with leadership, confidence and self-confidence, healing, hope, mercy and clarity and in releasing the negative conditions of passivity, doubt, futility, pessimism, hopelessness and confusion, both in the self and the world.

The Virtues are responsible for miracles and are able to beam out divine energy. Sometimes they are called 'shining ones' or 'brilliant ones'. Tradition says that the angels of the Ascension (of Jesus) were virtues. In Mahler's Eighth Symphony a chorus of angels lift Faustus's soul into the higher realm. He felt direct inspiration from the creative source for this symphony, and wrote to a friend, Willem Mengelberg: 'Imagine that the Universe bursts into song. We hear no longer human voices, but those of planets and suns which revolve'. The virtues work with group energy and they are working with all the spiritual groups that are now springing up. If you work in a meditation group or spiritual circle there is bound to be an angel for the group. As more groups come into being, there will be an inflow of spiritual energy into the planet, to raise vibrations. There are traditions that expect a new golden age to come into being—even that we are at the beginning of it. Although if you look around the world you might doubt this, there are many small spiritual groups springing up and ordinary people are gaining confidence to work directly with angelic and spiritual energy instead of through the established religions.

They say:

> Be confident in the words that we say to you and as you hear them, rather than in the words you read in books. This is the main message in your book *Hand in Hand with Angels*—that each one of you can make your own connection to us. You don't need mediums or any other authority except your own confidence.

The internet also provides new possibilities to connect with people all over the world who have similar interests, for there are many groups who meditate at the same time using the internet. In this upsurge of spiritual interest we may detect the influence of the virtues.

Call on Raphael, whose name means ' the medicine of God', or 'God heals,' when you want to work with the virtues. He will help you to keep on your spiritual path and act as a guide. The virtues enable people to live and work with righteousness, strength of will, gratitude, grace, courage and miracles. They will help to release the negative habits of arrogance, envy, resentment, ingratitude and temptation. They are thought to be the miracle workers and will suspend physical laws to allow the impossible.

The Powers keep the records of humanity, the collective history. They are like heavenly caretakers. Angels of birth and death are powers. They can absorb spiritual energy just like a tree absorbs sunlight and then send us a vision of a world spiritual network and the highest ideals that we can aspire to. In the same way that we have physical organs like heart, lungs, liver, kidneys, etc., so the different world religions are like different organs in the spiritual body of the planet. Powers govern universal laws like gravity, magnetism and similar. Camael, 'He who sees God', is the power to ask to help you when your life needs strength and determination. Call on powers for help when divine justice is needed, for inner strength and energy, decision-making, patience and justice. They will help to overcome weakness, thoughts of revenge, aggression, selfishness and egocentricity.

In ancient art, powers were depicted as lightning bolts.* How fascinating that the famous boy wizard, Harry Potter, has a lightning flash on his forehead. Can it be that the powers also communicate with us through stories?

The third sphere of angels is composed of those who act as heavenly messengers. They are the principalities, archangels and angels. The Principalities are the guardian angels of large groups, nations, governments, leaders, cities and even multinational organizations. Today, some people call them integrating angels. They hold the highest vision of a nation or organization and inspire people to work towards that vision, to work for the highest good. There is an angel that holds the vision of a unified planet in its heart. Whenever groups meditate for world peace or work for the highest good, they are tuning in to this angelic vision. It encourages the power of positive thought and is behind the increasing interest in self-help and New Age books, which inspire the use of affirmations and positive thought, so that people begin to create hope instead of negativity in all its aspects.

Everyone is familiar with the Archangels. Gabriel, for one, was the heavenly messenger who traditionally appeared to Mary to tell her about the birth of Jesus. He appeared to Mohammed and inspired the writing of the Koran. His name

Ask Your Angels, by Alma Daniel, Timothy Wyllie and Andrew Ramer.

means 'God is my Strength'. He inspires writers and all who teach the higher spiritual truths.

Archangel Michael's special day is on September 29th, Michaelmas, and Michaelmas daisies are named after him. His name means 'He who is as God'. Raphael is associated with healing and his name means 'God is healing'. Uriel (Auriel) is an angel of light. His name means 'God is my Light' or, as we have seen, 'Fire of God'. He is often seen with a flame burning in the palm of his hand. The archangels oversee human endeavour and sometimes are looked on as overlighting angels. Gabriel, Michael, Raphael and Uriel are the best known of the archangels.

Angels are the last of the hierarchy and are the ones we are most familiar with. They are the ones who work most closely with people and they have different roles. We know guardian (personal) angels the best. They are not only guardians, but are also spiritual guides, inspiring us to the highest we can achieve. However, do not confuse angels with spirit guides, who have had a human incarnation at some time. Everyone has a guardian angel as well as a spirit guide.

There are other traditions of angels as well as this one from Pseudo-Dionysius.

Standing just to one side of the Christian tradition the Essenes, an ancient spiritual community who lived before and after the birth of Jesus, had a tradition of a daily angelic meditation.* In the mornings, these were dedicated to the Earthly Mother and the Angels of Earth, Life, Joy, Sun, Water and Air, while in the evenings they were focused on the Angels of Eternal Life, Creative Work, Peace, Power, Love, Wisdom and the Heavenly Father. The Essenes believed that companionship with angels and the invisible energies of the universe bring health. They had meditations that brought awareness of the different energies which flow from nature. The meditations brought into awareness the organs and centres within the human body and aura that can receive those energies, and bring about a connection between the organs and centres and the corresponding forces, so that they can

*The Gospel of the Essenes, by Edmond Bordeaux Szekely

be absorbed, controlled and used. They thought that people could learn to live intuitively and in harmony with their inner guidance by meditating with angels. The Essenes believed that there would come a time in world history when so many people would work for the light that they would outnumber those who perpetuated war and violence. Then peace would come to the world and the universe. This sounds so familiar to us today when we are surrounded by books and workshops about health, abundance and spiritual development and Internet sites for prayer and spiritual discovery.

There is also renewed interest today in the Hebrew mystical tradition, represented by the Kabbalah, and there are ten archangels associated with it. These are Sandalphon (Trust), Auriel (Tenderness), Gabriel (Change), Raphael (Healing), Hanael (Blood), Michael (Sunshine), Samael (Adversity), Zadkiel (Wealth), Zaphkiel (Love), Raziel (Wisdom), Metatron (Judgment).* Note the rather different way the names are ascribed, compared to the tradition I have given.

There are many angelic traditions, and in the last few years there have been many books and workshops about angels. It is important not to get caught up in the differing and sometimes complicated traditions about angels, but rather to use meditation as a personal aid to build a bridge to the angels that you would like to work with and contact. Be confident that with pure selfless intentions you can contact the angelic world and develop experience in understanding your own intuition and guidance, and that you can work with your personal angels in the way that is right for your own spiritual unfoldment and development.

* *The Angels' Script,* by Theolyn Cortens

Seeing Angels

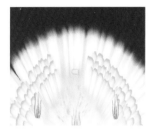

I have already suggested that people tend to dismiss their visions and dreams as 'only imagination', and yet imagination is the doorway to another world. The word 'imagine' means to make or receive an internal image or picture. We use this gift of imagination to create everything we ever do. Whatever we plan, whether it's a career, decorating a room, planning a holiday or merely the weekly shopping, it begins in our minds. The act of writing a shopping list, or visiting a DIY store or a travel agent, or planning the right training for the work we want to do, all begins in the imagination. The pictures in our minds are the doorways to achievement. The spiritual teachings of the world remind us that we are made in the image of Father–Mother God or the Source of All-That-Is, but in the way we create our lives we are co-creators. The pictures in our minds are the ways we create the things we want. The spiritual teacher, White Eagle, has said:

> 'The reason you are all afraid of imagination is that you do not understand what it truly is … whenever you see pictures (in your mind), whenever you imagine, you are seeing clearly, you are using the faculty of spiritual clairvoyance…. What you must do then, is to bring the will into action.' *Meditation*, by Grace Cooke

He also says that the only thing to fear is fear itself, so when we let gloomy pictures and ideas fill our thoughts, we can bring them into reality. There are other ways akin to meditation of becoming aware of spirit or angelic communication, such as clairaudience, claircognizance and clairsentience.

In clairaudience, you can hear spiritual teaching inside your mind. This is not to be confused with hearing voices that instruct you to do anything against your own conscience. Whatever guidance comes through clairaudience, or any other spiritual guidance, should be tested with good sense. Wait for the same guidance three times altogether and then always take careful consideration. Make sure it is the right thing to do before taking action. Divine guidance is always loving. Ask your guardian angel for help with making the right decisions.

Claircognizance is inspiration through thoughts. Notice the thoughts that regularly come into your mind. Don't dismiss your thoughts as nonsense, especially if they come again and again. Every new direction in life comes intuitively or through dreams. Many scientific discoveries have resulted from dreams. Claircognizance also shows itself as an inner knowing. You know something without knowing how you know it. It is often confirmed by the things people say to you or what you might read in books or hear on radio or television.

Spiritual guidance may also occur as physical or emotional feelings, known as clairsentience. We need to acknowledge the guidance that we receive from the way we feel about things. Sometimes we make a decision that might be right when viewed logically, yet we feel unhappy or depressed about it. We call that a gut feeling. A good decision is one that makes the heart sing, as long as it doesn't hurt another person.

The world of spirit is all around us and communicates with us through mental pictures or dreams. We cannot see this world with our normal sight as it vibrates more quickly, just like the patterns and colours on a spinner, which we played with as children, changed as its speed changed. So the angels communicate with us in our imagination, daydreams and dreams, through symbols and imagery, through light and colour. Visualization is always a safe way to communicate with angels. It helps us to go to their world.

We have deliberately chosen different styles of artwork to show the ways that people might visualize angels, for each person does so in their own unique way. Morgan's illustrations are not intended to match the text precisely, but to let you, the reader, use your own creative imagination. If you have artistic talents, keep a little sketchbook and try and jot down what you think angels look like every time you get inspiration. Even a squiggle is worthwhile. One of the reasons we have chosen some very abstract forms is so that—even if you do not think you are very good at art—you feel encouraged to play with colours and see where they take you.

KEEP A MEDITATION JOURNAL OR EVEN A SKETCHBOOK!

Find a beautiful notebook that inspires you to write down your meditations. I like to write with different coloured pens. If you like drawing, you can illustrate it—or keep your own angel sketchbook. Alternatively, keep a journal on your computer. Make it as interesting or beautiful as you can.

Your Regular Angel Meditation

Find a quiet place to sit where you will not be disturbed. Turn off the phone or put the answerphone on. If you like to burn essential oils, a good choice is either frankincense or sandalwood, as they have been used in meditation for thousands of years. These oils quieten the thoughts and help to take us out of the head mind, which is so persistent. For other ideas, see my book, ESSENTIAL OILS AND MEDITATION (London, Polair Publishing, 2007). Fresh flowers or plants are also good to have. I like to have a single rose in front of me when I meditate. It is a symbol for the heart chakra. Taking our attention into the heart centre (chakra) helps us to get out of the head mind with its at times intrusive thoughts.

Sit comfortably—in a chair or on the floor in a yoga meditation position if you prefer. Close your eyes and begin to breathe gently and smoothly. When you feel centred and relaxed, focus your breath into the centre of your chest. Feel your chest rising and falling with your breath. Then, after a few breaths, begin to imagine a bright light, like a sun or a star, in your heart centre (chakra) at the centre of your chest. With each breath, it begins to grow and expand until it fills your chest and then surrounds you with light. This process of filling and surrounding yourself with light protects you as you prepare to meditate. Light symbolizes Father–Mother God, the Source of All-That-Is and the Angels of Light.

Continue with your chosen meditation, whether it is the one described overleaf ('Meet your personal angel in the rose garden') or one from elsewhere in the book.

When you are ready to close your meditation, focus again on your breathing. Be aware once again of your physical body and breathe more deeply. There are a number of ways to do this and if you are an experienced meditator, you will know them. If you are not, try this: listen to the sounds around you; rub the palms of your hands together to bring your attention back to your everyday feelings, and then cup them over your eyes. Feel the warmth coming into you from your hands. Blink behind your hands and then open your eyes and have a good stretch. Make sure you are grounded again by visualizing roots going from the soles of your feet into the earth. Have a glass of cool water and walk around the room, feeling the ground beneath your feet.

If you're keeping a meditation journal, remember to write up your experience afterwards. The instructions on this page can be used each time you meditate.

Meditation: Meet your personal

Visualize yourself bathed in brilliant shining light.* This light not only surrounds you, but fills you. It protects you from all harm. As you continue to breathe deeply and slowly, you realize that every atom and cell of your whole being is sparkling and radiating light. You feel as if you are filled with millions of sparkling, radiating suns as every cell of your whole being becomes alive with light, even the genes in the DNA itself. This light protects you. Begin each day by visualizing it surrounding you and filling you wherever you go. It can also surround your house, car, friends and family, keeping them safe and protected. The white light is also the Source of All-That-Is, the Creator. You can do this breathing every day before going to work or whenever you need to.

As you become used to the light, you see a path of light ahead of you. Walk along the path, where it leads. You come to a beautiful park. Feel soft green grass beneath your bare feet. The sun is shining and you hear the sound of birds singing. Inhale the perfume of the flowers, brought to you on a soft gentle breeze.

Continue walking along the grassy path until you come to a rose garden. Here there are beds of roses of many different colours. There is a path with arches of white roses over it. As you walk along it, you smell their scent.

When you come to the end of the path, it opens out into a circular arbour of white roses climbing up white trellises. A circle of soft green grass with white benches all around is inside the rose arbour. Go and sit on one of the benches. You feel excited because you know you are going to meet your special angel, one that you have known for many years but can't quite remember! It is your guardian angel.

ANGEL IN THE ROSE GARDEN...

Feel the light that radiates from your heart centre as it begins to expand again and call your special angel to you. Send out a vibration of love and light, knowing that your angel will feel it and come to meet you. The angel will only come when you call.

Imagine how the angel looks. What colour is it wearing? Does it look as you would imagine it or not? Can you only see light and colour? Some people only see beautiful eyes, or coloured light. There might be the scent of perfume like roses or lilies or violets. Don't have any expectations, just accept what you see. Be confident that it is not 'just imagination'. You know that this angel has been with you throughout the ages, through many lives, and knows you exactly as you are and loves and admires you for your courage in volunteering for life on earth with all its challenges. Know that you are loved and supported, whatever you do.

Invite the angel to come and sit beside you. Ask its name. Don't worry if you don't hear it the first time. Whatever you hear will be confirmed in some way in everyday life. There might be a beautiful perfume or colour. Take note of what the angel looks like, so you will know it again. It might give you a symbol that will remind you of it, so you know it is there when you see the symbol. You might see a crystal, a star, a shell, a ring, or a flower. Thank the angel for supporting you and say goodbye.

To do this meditation, use the process described on p. 27. To remember the meditation in a way that you can use it another time without having to read the text, you can read it through several times or record it into an audio recorder. Conclude your meditation in the way described.

What might your special (guardian) angel look like? People see angels in all sorts of different ways. Some see an angel as pure light and colour, with beautiful piercing eyes. Sometimes they can appear as in medieval art or as in the Victorian pictures that are familiar to us. They might look just like an ordinary person. One day, when I was facilitating an angel course, I took the participants through a visualization to see a special angel who would be with them to help them. I was surprised when I saw a special angel for me as well, because I don't tune in for myself when facilitating a workshop. But there he was, very large, dressed in motorbike leathers. 'My name is Kenneth', he said. 'I am always with you when you

HOW TO WORK WITH ANGELS

1. Meditation using creative visualization is a safe way to contact spirit guides and angels. Imagination is the key to clairvoyance. Other forms of contacting them are hearing (clairaudience) and knowing (claircognizance).

2. When you meet a guide or angel in the scene you create in your mind's eye, you need to invite them in. The 'doorway' is on your side. Spiritual law is that they cannot interfere with your freewill until you invite them to help you.

3. To protect yourself from mischievous spirits, you can ask three times, 'Are you from God and All–Light?'. It is spiritual law that they must leave after the third time of asking if they are not. Visualizing yourself surrounded by light is also protective.

4. Ask your angel to show you a symbol that will always be associated with you both. They can show you it three times as a means of identification. It will be something simple like a rose or cross or star, something that is especially meaningful to you.

5. When you want or need to contact your unseen friends,

go out by yourself. My work is to protect you'. He was very insistent that he was not to be called Ken.

I would never have imagined that an angel of light would look like a biker, but there you are! I know I am always safe. A long time later, I asked him to show me what he is like as a heavenly angel, an angel of light. He showed me that he is enormous, as tall as the room we were in. I don't visualize angels with robes or wings. I see their light and colours and usually their eyes. His light was all shades of violet, lilac and amethyst. He is definitely an angel of light, working on the violet ray. If anyone noticed him with me in the city, they would see him in his biking leathers!

make an 'appointment' with them, just as you would with any friend. You wouldn't be phoning or dropping in on them at inconvenient times or expecting it from them. People can fall into the mistake of being flattered when woken up at all hours for 'spirit messages'.

6. Remember you always have freewill. Never do anything suggested to you that conflicts with commonsense or with the law. If you ever hear voices that suggest you do bad things, stop working alone and find a safe meditation group or development group.

7. Always make sure you are firmly grounded and centred after meditation. A good way to do this is to imagine roots going from the soles of your feet into the ground to keep you earthed. They are like roots of light that enable you to move freely but keep you from dreaminess. If you do feel 'spaced out', drink mineral water with 'rescue remedy' (the Bach flower remedy, or its equivalent in another system, such as Julian Barnard's Five Flower Remedy), or clematis flower remedy. These remedies bring you out of dreamy states. If you need to, then go for a walk or take some physical exercise. If the dreaminess continues to affect you, stop working alone and find a training course where you can work under supervision and with the help of a teacher.

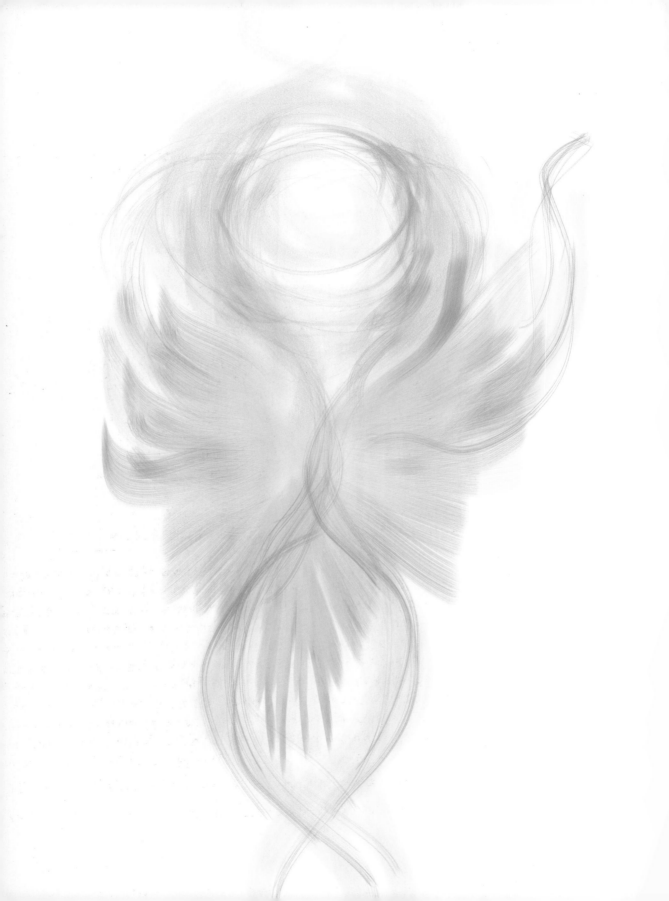

2.

Our Partnership with Angels

A NGELS are everywhere. Frequently aware of them as I am, I one day heard the words that follow. (I shall have more of these 'intuitive listenings' to share as the book continues.)

> We are all around you. We listen to your meditations and talk to you. We are at your spiritual development groups and the yoga classes that retain a spiritual element, in the way that the ancient yogis taught, for we taught the rishis of old. They opened their inner vision, saw us and communed with us, as you do. We listen to your spiritual discussions and draw your attention to the messages on the angel cards you draw at our guidance and inspiration. Take every opportunity to talk about us so that the partnership between angels and people becomes strong.

I think people and angels were always meant to work together. As we have seen, in ancient myths and legends angels and otherworldly beings were always there to help people in difficulty. We have the remnant of these ancient tales in folk stories and even pantomime. Angels say, 'The first essential on your side is a belief in our existence'.* Once we believe that angels are there, we are more open to their help. The handle of the door to unseen worlds is indeed on our side. We see and hear them in the ways they communicate with us. Sometimes these are very subtle, sometimes very noticeable. People often dismiss things as coincidence or imagination, but it is not

* *The Brotherhood of Angels and of Men*, by Geoffrey Hodson, p. 9

always so. Humans have freewill, freedom of choice, freedom to choose right action or not, so we need to ask for help when we need it.

There are too many stories about people who are miraculously saved from danger for them to be dismissed as coincidence. What we call coincidence is the law of synchronicity in action, and when you look back over events in your life, you can see how things often work out for the better. It's the help of the angels, who will assist when they are needed. If we choose to work consciously with angels, we could make great changes in the world, changes for the better. The angels themselves tell us that the first task is to banish discord and ugliness from the world, and when people and angels work together, there will be a golden age,* as so many ancient traditions promise. So we can turn the handle of that door and invite angels into our lives.

How can we work consciously with the angels to make the world a more beautiful place? The first step is to use the thoughts and pictures in our minds to create beauty. Every time we find ourselves thinking a dreary or depressing thought, we can change the mental picture. We can change our minds. If you are afraid of something that might happen, visualize the event in your mind turning out well. Create pictures in your mind that show what you want to happen. If you are not a 'visual' type or think you don't have a very vivid imagination, you can write a daily diary or forecast, or plan goals you want to achieve.

One way in which humans were made in the image of the Source of All-That-Is is that we can choose our thoughts. It can be a hard struggle at times, but practising regular meditation and using affirmations as we work with our personal angel are helpful techniques. It's best not to watch too much violence on films and TV, or read too many depressing stories, especially just before bedtime as these can influence our dreams. We do need to be aware of world events to know where we need to send healing help, but we do not need to

*See, for instance, *The Brotherhood of Angels and of Men*, Geoffrey Hodson, just quoted

HAND IN HAND WITH ANGELS

become overwhelmed by what we see and hear so that we get upset and fearful. We need not always be reading or watching about these things. We don't have to be dragged down into depression by the negative stories and news that fill the press or the media. We do not need to dwell on unhappy thoughts or our fears, whatever they are. The late Wilfred Clarke, who founded the Friends of Yoga Society (FRYOG), was talking to an old lady one day. She said to him, 'You know, I've had many worries in my life, but most of them never happened.'

We can work with angels by using pictures in our minds (visualization) and words (affirmations, which combine visualization with thought power). If we study ancient and modern traditions this secret about the power of thought can be found. In her book, *The Game of Life and How to Play It*, Florence Scovel Shinn points out how to use the ancient secrets of the Old and New Testaments to work with God. *Whatever a man soweth that shall he also reap.* This means that whatever you send out, including your thoughts, will return to you. In the Holy Bible we read, *Carefully guard your thoughts because they are the source of true life.** In other words, your life is shaped by your thoughts.

The way we use this idea nowadays is through the use of affirmations. These are positive statements that we can make to ourselves that influence our thoughts and feelings. They are a part of the ancient yoga tradition of positive thinking and were called a *sankalpa*, or resolution. They are used in deep relaxation or meditation. Swami Satyananda Saraswati, in his book *Yoga Nidra*, says that the resolve (affirmation) should be kept very simple, should be stated three times in a positive manner during relaxation and it is bound to come true.† The reason that affirmations are used in relaxation and meditation is that in that state we are accessing deeper mental states, deeper states in the unconscious mind. Withdrawing the senses into deeper and deeper states of relaxation enables the practitioner to begin to overcome old bad habits of thought and action. Since relaxation arises out of trust, when you are relaxed your

*Galatians 6 : 7; Proverbs 4 : 23
†*Yoga Nidra*, Swami Satyananda Saraswati, p. 93

affirmation is much less likely to contain a hidden fear. Also, the mind is less likely to argue with the affirmations.

Emile Coué (1857–1926), a French pharmacist, was the pioneer in the use of affirmations in the early part of the twentieth century. He stated that all of our thoughts become reality. He believed the power of the imagination was stronger than willpower. Thinking sad thoughts can create more generalized feelings of unhappiness, and depression. If you think anxious thoughts, you feel tense, and tension increases unless you notice it and relax. He recommended that his patients should get into a comfortable relaxed position before going to bed or in bed before sleep, close their eyes and relax all of their muscles. He encouraged them to repeat, twenty times, the affirmation made famous by him, 'Every day in every way I'm getting better and better'.

Popular modern authors who write on the use of affirmations include Louise Hay, author of *You Can Heal Your Life*, and Shakti Gawain, who wrote *Creative Visualization*. Shakti Gawain thinks that visualization is a form of energy that creates life and life's happenings. Everything is energy and we create our world with the mind. As we saw earlier, the Creator, Source of All That Is, works through angels, who are His–Her messengers. We can ask for angelic help when we need to heal our lives and using visualization techniques and affirmations is a safe way to work with angels and brings extra strength to our visions.

An affirmation needs to be stated in the present tense so it is attracted into the 'now'. In the Native American tradition there is a belief in 'the field of plenty'.* Here the thought-forms exist to provide all we ever need in the physical world. To call these ideas into reality, we need a grateful heart. Thought always precedes form. So each morning and at convenient times during the day, we can call on the Light (God) by picturing our needs and thanking the angels of all light for bringing them into reality. When we act on the thoughts and good ideas in our minds, they start to act in the physical world, which includes our own bodies.

A good affirmation to begin the day is the one opposite. Use

*See *Sacred Path Cards*, by Jamie Sams

HAND IN HAND WITH ANGELS

> Infinite Spirit, Beloved Mother/Father God, Thank you for this new day and all the beautiful things that come to me. Today is filled with good and I am filled with joy, happiness and success.

your own favourite term for God, such as the Source. Visualize your special angel by your side as you say this and as you go through the day, helping you and guiding you to do the right things and make the right decisions. Sometimes you might get an insight during meditation. You might get a gut feeling or intuition. You might hear a voice. Always be prepared to follow your vision, to live your dream, providing no one is hurt by what you do and you are not avoiding your worldly duties.

Accept that the All-Light/All-Love has given you everything you will ever need. Just begin to work with it and, like the yeast makes the bread rise, all that you ever hope to be will expand little by little until you *are* all that you *hope* to be.

It seems that angels are coming closer and closer to human beings. There are more and more books and songs about angels. The shops are filled with angel cards and ornaments. There are even shops that are completely dedicated to angel gifts and ideas. But in reality, it's people who are growing closer and closer to angels. Angels have always surrounded us. People are opening up to the idea of angels being around them. There are not so many people who dismiss angels as imaginary.

There are self-help books and methods which help people to banish ugliness and discord from the world. This is what angels are looking for in humans and every effort made to weed out negative thinking and bad habits bring the angels nearer and nearer to us. Many self-help books are available and there are many workshops devoted to healing, self-development and related issues. As people work on ways of clearing old issues, old thoughts, old memories, it's as if they're pulling old thorns out. Then they can get to the beautiful layers underneath that are like a flower bulb. As each old layer is stripped away, they get nearer and nearer to the beautiful flower within. By watering that bulb with love (loving themselves) it will grow into a beautiful flower—a white lily, with golden edges on each petal and with a beautiful perfume. Another way of looking at it is as if old grimy windows are being cleaned. When they are dusty and smeared with grime, the light can't get in and you can't see out of them. Everything looks misty and unclear. Once the windows are washed and polished, everything looks clear, bright and shiny and more and more light comes in. When you are open to seeing things in a new way, new ideas become more acceptable, more obvious.

An important way to make room for angels in your life is to begin to make all your surroundings as uncluttered and beautiful as possible. By creating a special corner for meditation, affirmations and healing prayers, gradually, over time, the area spreads until one day you may be able to have a small room entirely devoted to meditation and healing. Eventually, every room can have special objects and ornaments. There may be beautiful bowls or large shells containing potpourri and crystals on shelves and windowsills. A special effort is made to keep each area clean and freshly decorated so that there is an ethos and atmosphere in which spiritual energy develops. Put flowers and candles and some incense on a small table and play some soothing music to help to 'tune in' with the light. The best way to change the world is to begin with oneself and the surroundings where we live. The same ideas would work whether you lived in a bedsit or mansion, a forest hut or Himalayan cave. Your surroundings can still be clean, tidy and uncluttered, with the spiritual objects that you like to use to inspire your connection to angels.

It is also a good idea to light a candle each day to the angels of the house. Every home has its own guardian angels. If you acknowledge their presence they will co-operate with you and help to protect the home. Below is a prayer which can be used daily when the candle is lit.

> Angels of God, the guardians here, to whom His–Her love commits us dearly, always be at my (our) side today, to light and guard, to help, heal and guide. Thank you for guarding this house, and us, night and day and keeping it safe when we're in, out and away. Bless all who live here, all who come here.

Angels, or 'light beings' are very significant in the work of the one known as 'the Bulgarian Master', Peter Deunov (Beinsa Douno), who gave us the sacred dance known as Paneurhythmy. Here are two of his prayers or 'formulas', rather like the one I have just set out, to say when we arrive in a new place and when we leave. They are normally said three times.*

O kindly luminous beings, guardians of this place,
be hospitable with us, and may God bless you.

O kindly luminous beings, guardians of this place,
thank you for your hospitality, and may God bless you.

Burning essential oils in a lamp can also improve the atmosphere and environment of the home. These oils help to clear away the smell of cooking or cigarettes and make the atmosphere pleasant and welcoming. Good oils to clear household smells are cedarwood, cypress, eucalyptus, lavender, any of the lemon-scented oils like lemon itself, citronella, may chang or lemon grass, and rosemary. Other oils generate the brain waves of meditation. One of the special benefits of frankincense, lavender or sandalwood oil is to slow the brain waves and heart rate. When we are in a calm mood, it is easier to meditate and draw close to our guardian angels.

Music is also an important way of keeping the home energy positive and attracting angels. They can come nearer when the energy is harmonious. Loud, discordant music creates the wrong energy. The world we live in has become very noisy and it seems almost impossible to get away from the noise of traffic, aircraft, neighbours and the busy city. Sometimes the radio, TV or music centre seems to be kept permanently on. Although it is in the quietness we can contact angels best,† playing relaxing music in the background stops the distraction of outside noises. Geoffrey Hodson wrote in 1932 that invoking guardian angels will surround our homes with love, protection and blessing. However, they do appeal for

*From *Prayers and Songs*, by Beinsa Douno
†*Spiritual Unfoldment 2*, by White Eagle, pp. 33-4

more quietness, harmony and spirituality. It seems we have created an almost impassable barrier of noise and materialism between the angels and ourselves. It is certainly noisier now than when Hodson was writing in the thirties.·

Music is a personal taste, of course, but in my view Baroque music, like Vivaldi and Albinoni, creates the right atmosphere—or some of the slower passages of Mozart. My favourite music for meditation that brings the angels close is New Age music. New Age music is written especially to create the slow brain waves that enable the meditative mood that insulates against outside noise. It also helps to prevent troublesome thoughts from interfering with our meditations. Music and burning meditative essential oils can both create the special atmosphere that enables angels to draw close. My own book, *Essential Oils and Meditation*, may help here.

Similar ideas can be used in subtle ways in the place where you work. Usually there is not much scope for anything elaborate, but a simple focal point on a desk, such as a crystal which might serve as a paperweight can help to change the energy of the workplace to one of beauty and harmony. Rose quartz is a crystal that has special affinity with the angelic kingdom. It is known as the love stone. It is very good for the energy of the heart centre.

A few years ago, one of my friends asked if there was a crystal I could recommend for a colleague of hers who had had a heart attack. When the colleague returned to work, she caused a great deal of unhappiness in the department because of her constant misery and grumbling. It got so bad that people were trying to avoid her—which, of course, made her even more miserable. I suggested rose quartz and my friend gave it to her colleague for a birthday present. She reported back to me that in a short time the woman had become cheerful and friendlier and the atmosphere was completely different. Rose quartz has been used to good effect to clear a bad atmosphere at work. A piece can be kept on the desk as an ornament or even in the drawer, out of sight. Rose quartz is also the crystal to be kept in the relationship corner of the home or living room, if you

* *The Coming of the Angels*, by Geoffrey Hodson

work with feng shui. It is a good stone to keep in the bedroom, to keep the atmosphere restful and harmonious.

All buildings and businesses have their guardian angels. Through the power of creative imagination, these great beings will work in co-operation with us as we try to do our work responsibly. When going to meetings, visualize the angel of the particular business or company. You don't need to know the angel's name, although if you are very intuitive you might hear one. Just visualize the appropriate angel (e.g., accountancy, travel, teaching, medicine etc.), and visualize peace and harmony and the best outcome for the meeting. A suitable affirmation is

Angel of (e.g., accountancy)—thank you for a perfect and harmonious outcome to this meeting. This is now released for the highest good of all concerned.

When there is discord in a building or office, visualize the angels of the people and the businesses involved bringing a harmonious resolution that is good for all the people involved. Suitable affirmations could be

Thank you for a beneficial outcome for (..........) or All is in Divine Order.

The same thing can be done when travelling to prevent being caught up in road rage or with quarrelsome people. The great protecting angel with responsibility for protecting the earth is Archangel Michael. Keep a small picture of him in the car or briefcase, hidden in one of the compartments. Whenever I travel, I use Archangel Michael's prayer. I suggest saying it three times:

Lord Michael to the right, Lord Michael to the left.
Lord Michael before, Lord Michael behind,
Lord Michael above, Lord Michael below,
Lord Michael, Lord Michael, wherever I go.

I used this prayer once when I felt nervous driving on a quiet country road. A large white van was driving far too close for my liking, tailgating me. I couldn't go any faster and the road was too narrow and winding for it to overtake. Before I had finished thinking the prayer, the van had fallen back and was soon completely out of sight. I had not noticed any lanes or farms where it might have turned off.

Every garden has a guardian angel, known as the guardian of the land. It looks after all the nature spirits and living things that have made the garden their home. The guardian angel is better able to work when the owners do not use chemical pesticides. A garden can be simple and have herbs, shrubs and flowers that attract butterflies and bees and other helpful insects. Some people have 'green fingers', a gift with plants. The plants respond to the love of the gardener and the pleasure they find in it. The whole of life responds to loving energy and the angels of nature are able to co-operate with gardeners who love working with plants. Angels are concerned with the formation of physical life and the life of plants improves with co-operation between people and the angels.

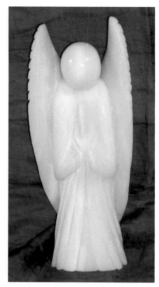

Mangano Calcite Angel
imported by Geo Art

'It is quite possible for the gardener or farmer so to attune himself to the angels and fairy kingdom as to work in co-operation and partnership with them to produce the very finest and best results'.

White Eagle, *Spiritual Unfoldment 2*

Keeping statues of angels in the garden will remind you of them. It is also a good idea to put large crystals in each corner of the garden and in special places. If you have a garden, one thing you can do to consciously become aware of angels is to meditate in the garden at the start of each season. Use your inner vision (imagination, if you like) and 'see' the angels in the garden. You can put a pinch of sacred smudge (white sage) in each corner of the garden to represent the four directions and the four mighty archangels traditionally associated with them. East represents spring, the dawn and Archangel Raphael. The south represents summer, midday and Archangel Michael. The west represents autumn, the evening and Archangel

When planting vegetables, seeds or plants, surround them with sage (smudge) and thank the nature spirits and angels for their help in growing healthy and sustaining plants and vegetables.

Mentally talk to them as you would talk to your friends. Cover the smudge with soil when you finish the planting. If you live in a flat, you can do the same thing with your houseplants, putting the sage into the plant pot.

ANGELIC CO-OPERATION IN ACTION

The famous Findhorn Garden was conceived in the 1960s as an experiment to find the way that angels, nature spirits and people could work together. The recommended process derived from Findhorn is:

1. Recognize that angels and nature spirits (devas) do exist and give them love and thanks.
2. Through thought-power, ask for their help. Know that they are there and speak to them silently or aloud, thanking them for their help.
3. Pay special attention to your intuitive thoughts and feelings. You might not get direct guidance through a voice, but with a feeling of inner knowing about what to do. Notice what works and what doesn't and always work with what is successful.
4. Lovingly thank the angels and nature spirits.

Gabriel, while the north represents winter, night-time and Archangel Auriel. Do this at the winter and summer solstice and spring and autumn equinox and thank the archangels of the four directions and seasons for their help in nurturing the garden. Thank them for any benefits you want or have noticed. Remember that the future is drawn in from the 'field of plenty', the universe, and humbly and gratefully thank the angels in advance for what it is you would like to happen in the garden.

The white sage that you need is imported from America. European sage doesn't make good smudge or incense and it doesn't burn well. It is smoky and smells a lot. Rosemary or lavender can be dried and used as a cleansing herb. I haven't tried burning it as incense, but incenses are fun to make.*

The more things we can do to bring beauty and harmony into our lives, the easier it is for angels to come near and work with us. As the angels told the well-known writer about angels, Geoffrey Hodson, 'Discord and ugliness must vanish from the world; to remove it is our task and yours—but yours first'.†

*For more advice see the Polair Guide *Incense*, by Jennie Harding
† *The Coming of the Angels*, p. xxii

ATTUNEMENT ACTIVITIES

MAKING AN ANGEL TREASURE BOX
(BOX OF SECRETS) OR AN ANGEL VISION BOARD

A fun way to make it easy to work with angels is to make **an angel treasure box,** or box of secrets. Find a beautiful box of a size you like. It can be a gift box you find in a greetings card shop, or one you might have been given with presents in. It might already be decorated with shiny paper or you can decorate it yourself if you like craft work. It needs to be as beautiful and decorative as possible. In the box you can keep your favourite angel cards, angel ornaments and sprinkles, crystals and silk purses to keep them in, dried flowers, an essential oil or perfume, like rose, jasmine or orange blossom (neroli) that brings peace and happiness to you and enables angels to come closer.

In the box, keep a beautiful notebook with a decorated cover where you can write the affirmations you are working with. It's a good idea to spend a few minutes each day to work with the things you keep in the box. You might read some of your affirmations aloud, or write a new one you have thought of. You could do an angel reading for yourself with your cards. You could find a little book of affirmations or short readings that inspire you to keep in your treasure box. These things form part of the 'law of attraction', and its secret to success is persistence.

As an alternative to making a treasure box, make **an angel vision board**. Obtain a large piece of coloured card of the type that can be found in stationery suppliers. Gold is a good colour. Cut as large a circle as you can and divide it into four quarters. Label the quarters as follows: Business; Family and Friends; Spiritual; Fun. Then allow your creative abilities to run riot. Cut out pictures from magazines, photocopy or print from the Internet, copy your photos. Put them into the relevant sections of your treasure map or vision board all the things you dream of achieving. A good time to do it is on New Year's Day, or your birthday. Ask your angels for inspiration. (See my own for 2010, shown here.) You may also buy inexpensive pinboards from the supermarket and pin on your plans for a month, a week, or even your five-year plan.

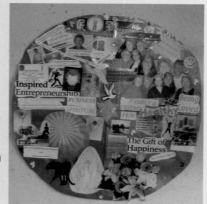

Meditation:
CALLING ANGELS TO YOUR HOME OR WORKPLACE

This meditation can be done mentally and from a distance, as it may not be possible to do anything at your workplace.

Sit in your favourite meditation pose and close your eyes and begin your meditation as on p. 27. With each breath, visualize yourself filling with light. See a light above you, like the sun, sending a shower of light all around you and within. Feel your chest filling with light. Send it all around your body until every atom and cell are radiating light like millions of tiny suns. See and feel rays of light radiating from your heart and filling the room where you are sitting. Fill your house or workplace with light and start to surround the external walls with a wall of light. Slowly visualize this wall of light moving around until the building is completely surrounded. Cover the windows and doors with light. Do the same with the floor and the roof, until the walls, floor and roof of the whole building are light. You can do this at a distance for a building, such as your workplace, where you would not be able to do it in private.

Once you have surrounded the building with light, begin to see the angels who are working with you in the home or workplace. Use all the power of your creative imagination and trust what you see. The angels might not look like the pictures you have seen. Sometimes they are seen as pure light and colour. You might see loving eyes looking at you. You might not see anything, but feel surrounded by love and support. Sometimes tears may come to your eyes; sometimes you might smell beautiful perfume or hear music. You might get goose bumps. If there are any problems in your home or work life, thank the angels for help with settling your problem in perfect and harmonious ways for the highest good of all concerned. Trust the angels to know what the highest good is, because they see with greater vision than we do.

You will know when this process is complete. Conclude the meditation according to the general instructions.

3.
Angels and Healing

Listen, listen, listen! We are everywhere. When you think you are overwhelmed, we are with you. We wait on you and wait for you to see us, to hear us. We will never interfere or interrupt, but open your inner vision and see us all around you. Open your ears, hear our soft whispers. Open your awareness and notice our messages that we send through friends, songs, books and films.

WHEN people are unwell, most of their thoughts are focused on getting better. Among the range of healing techniques we can call on is angelic attunement, and helping to administer healing are angels dedicated to doing so. They are always with us, but until we actually ask the angels of healing for help, they respect our freewill. Healers and therapists working in hospices and hospitals often talk about the angels they see when working with patients there. In my angel workshops I ask participants to share their angel stories as a way of helping them to realize that many people do have experiences of angels. An aromatherapist told about massaging terminally ill patients. She frequently saw colours and heard music around them.

A friend of mine, Geraldine, when in her seventies, told me the story printed overleaf, about the time her brother nearly died. It happened when she was about four years old, but she had never forgotten this incident.

Angels are always with us when we pray or meditate.

Geraldine's Story about Healing Angels

'My two brothers and I returned to London from Singapore with my mother, who was expecting her fourth baby, and our nanny. We were to begin our schooling. It was wintertime and there was an influenza epidemic. Inevitably we all went down with it. We were being cared for in the night nursery—a very large room, which easily took our three cots.

'On the night my angel came to visit, I knew, from all the commotion, that my elder brother was very ill indeed. Everyone, including the doctor, was clustering round his cot. I was miffed because I was hot, thirsty and frightened by all the comings and goings and all the shadows on the ceiling, but no one was taking any notice of me. Then I saw, bending over my brother's cot, a brilliantly shining lady with white light all around her, and wings. I tried to cry out, but no sound came and I remember putting my arms out to her, but that's all. I must have fallen asleep then. After that, we all slowly recovered, but no one could tell me who the lovely lady was and said I'd been dreaming. But I knew that wasn't so. Ever since then, I've sought my angel but I've never seen her again—though I thought I saw a hint of her smile when my twenty-two-month-old nephew was dying and I held him in my arms and he smiled.'

Children often see angels when they are young, but when told it is 'only imagination', they can lose the ability to do so or stop talking about them.

Angels work closely with healers, therapists and orthodox medical practitioners, inspiring them. It's always important to contact a doctor, but remember that working with him will always be healing angels. You don't have to count on him or her alone. Mary, an old lady in her eighties, tells the story of the time she broke her hip. It was a bank holiday and she went out for a walk. The pavement was uneven, and she caught her foot and fell. The ambulance came and took her to hospital. Luckily for her, the most experienced consultant in repairing broken hips was still in the hospital. He was having a half-hour

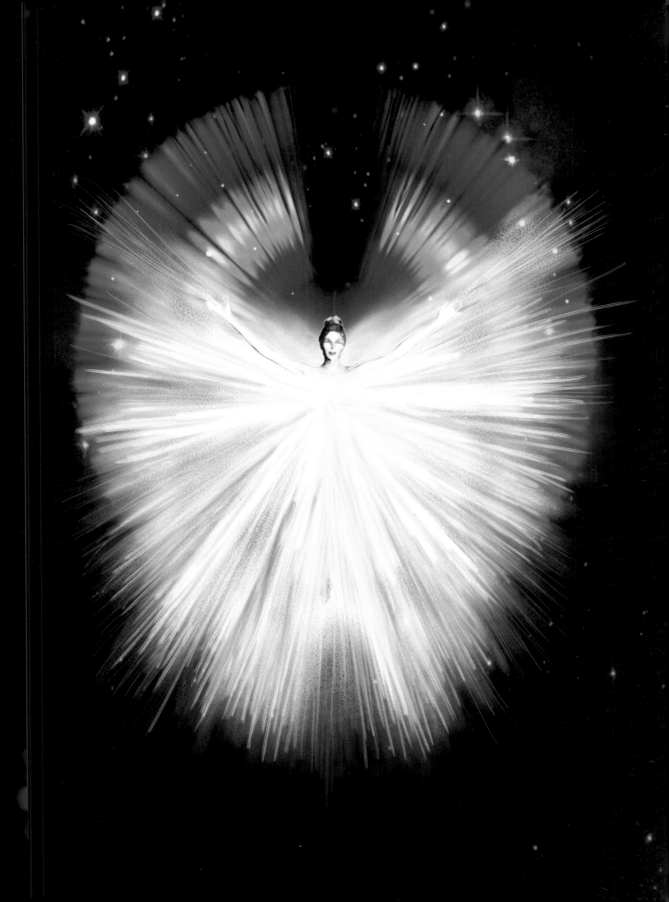

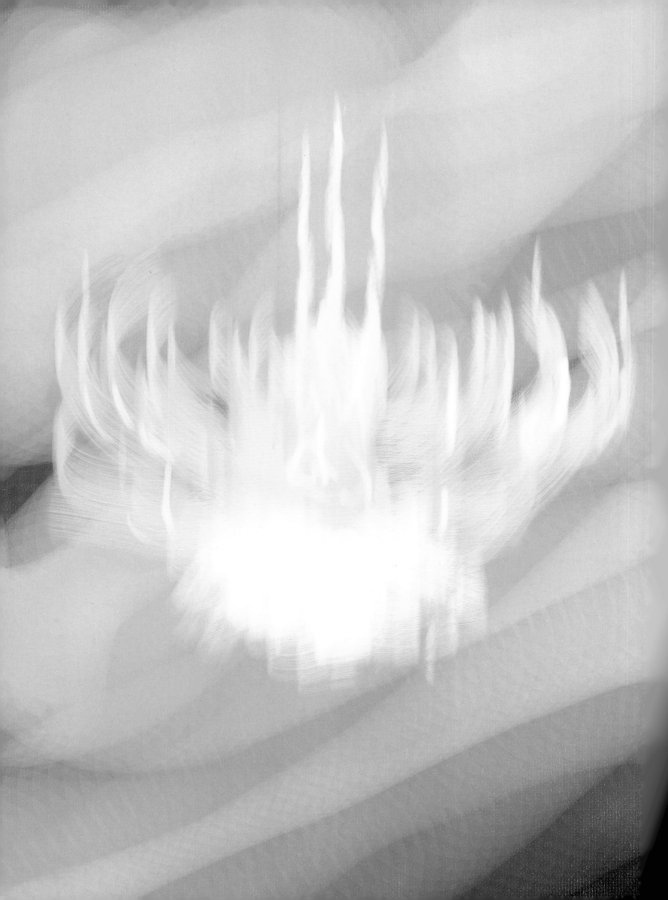

4.
Angels and the Essenes

THE ESSENES were a community that lived near the Dead Sea before and after the time of Jesus Christ. Some people today* say that they were practitioners of a tradition that was practised in the lost continent of Atlantis. They were very strict with their diet and way of life. They were vegetarians and lived communally, owning things in common. They believed they were surrounded by unseen energies, which they called angels, that would show them how to live in harmony with life. The Essenes would meditate upon an angel each morning when awakening and each evening before sleep. They would live their lives according to the insights they received in their meditations and believed this enabled them to live a more harmonious life. Edmond Bordeaux Szekely, who writes about them, calls their meditations 'communions'. The communions were a way of absorbing the qualities of the angels within the body, so that the Essenes made daily connections with the angels throughout their lives.†

The reasons for these communions were threefold. The first was to enable people to become aware of the different energies and vibrations that came from the universe and surrounded them, helping them to be healthier. The second was to gain an understanding of the physical organs and energy centres (chakras) of the body that can benefit from these energies. The third purpose was to make the connection between the organs and centres so that people could absorb, control and use each energy and vibration.

*e.g., the website www.arolotifar.com
†See *The Gospel of the Essenes*

Our different physical systems use vitamins, minerals and enzymes found in the food we eat, from the earth and in the environment, such as fresh air, sunshine and pure water. The ancients thought that life was defined by four elements: earth (the planet, the environment and provider of everything needed to sustain life); air (the breath and the thoughts); fire (the sunshine and love); water (for drinking and cleansing, representing the emotions and feelings).* There is quite a lot of discussion in the media at the moment about pesticides and herbicides and the way in which they can poison the environment and diminish the nutrients found in our food. There is a growing movement for eating organic food and growing one's own where possible.

The Essenes were not the only tradition to think that pure nourishment was important. Yogis also teach that diet and lifestyle are vital to physical, mental, emotional and spiritual health. They teach about *prana*, the invisible spiritual essence or life-force contained within the air we breathe. It is also found in pure healthy foods, preferably organic. The Chinese teach about chi energy, the life-force or spiritual energy, which can be absorbed through breath and the power of thought, as well as the foods we eat. In the Essene tradition the energies of the human body are described in terms of opposites just as in India and China: masculine/feminine and positive/negative (in the sense of magnetism and electricity), corresponding to *yin/yang* in the Chinese traditions and *ha/tha* in yoga.

If you are interested in your health and wellbeing and want to meditate with angels daily to improve it, you can use the Essene meditations to help you.

The morning meditations were based on the idea that the earth was our Earthly Mother. The Essenes thought of a person as a tree, with roots deep in the ground of the Earthly Mother The roots of the tree are her angels. The Earthly Mother provides all we need to live our daily lives, such as food and water, our clothes, our houses and our friends and

* See also chapter six, about the Four Archangels. When we talk about the elements they are not, of course, to be confused with the 112 elements of science.

family. Everything we need and use comes from the planet. The communions were regarded as a bridge between people and angels.

The branches of the tree are the angels of the Heavenly Father. These are the energies and vibrations of the invisible worlds. Many spiritual traditions say that as we fall asleep, the soul leaves the body to search for spiritual inspiration and truth in the world that we all return to at the end of life—that is, in the world of light or spirit world.

The communions with the angels of the Heavenly Father should take place just before sleep, just before going to bed or even in bed. They are the last thoughts before sleep. It is not good to watch negative films or the news at this juncture, as spiritual teachers tell us that the last thoughts before sleep influence the place the soul visits while the body is asleep.

The intention of the meditations is very important, as they should not be automatic. The intention should be meaningful and filled with enthusiasm and joy, not dead, like dead leaves that blow here and there wherever the wind takes them. Because the working week is so busy, these meditations need not be long. Five to ten minutes is probably long enough as long as the intention is clear and pure, so that you are thoroughly attuned to the energies of the daily angels. The angels were not given names, as it was felt they represented qualities that one should try to develop.

On the following fourteen pages, I have given my own interpretation of the Essene meditations, adapted for use today. Note that the tradition corresponds to the Jewish one, in which Saturday, not Sunday, is the day of rest, or Sabbath. The affirmations given in this section are my own, ones which I have used and found helpful.

Saturday Morning
The Earthly Mother

The first meditation, or communion, begins on Saturday morning. It is intended to bring unity between the body and the nutrients of the earth. It should be done as soon as you awake. On this and every morning, become aware that your body is waking up so that you can go about your daily tasks. As you wake up, breathe health and energy into your body. Feel yourself becoming one with the earth, who is like a mother in providing all our needs. She provides all the food we need, which grows in the rich soil of the Planet Earth.

WAKE UP TO LIFE!

Affirm:
Thank you for this new day.
The Earthly Mother and I are one.
All the health and strength I need come from her.
She cares for me and I do my best to care for her.

Breathe deeply and feel your lungs filling with life-giving energy. Surround yourself with light. Breathe it in and breathe it down into your body and out through your legs and feet into the ground, the Earthly Mother. As you look into the light, you see the beautiful form of the Earthly Mother. She looks like a goddess of nature, with long flowing hair and like your ideal picture of the perfect woman. She is dressed in robes of green, with the colours of flowers, herbs and grasses, cereals and food plants adorning her. On her head is a crown of flowers.

The earth is hers, and she will heal it from the pollution and exploitation that has been inflicted on it, but she tells you that she needs your help to do it. Every person who can live in a sustainable way to the best of their ability helps to heal the planet. She asks you what is the best thing you can do so you tell her what you are able to do. She radiates even more light to you, which strengthens and sustains your ideas. Thank her for her blessing. Then she leaves and you feel encouraged and strengthened by her.

Saturday Evening
THE ANGEL OF ETERNAL LIFE

The Saturday evening communion was an important one. The Essenes meditated about the Cosmos and the laws of the universe. They contemplated the ways they were part of the whole of creation and what they could do to enhance it.

Breathe calmly and slowly, and use these affirmations.

> I fill myself with light.
> I am one with the Heavenly Father and Earthly
>   Mother and with all of life.
> Light fills my whole being,
> I am released from all fears and worries.

MEET THE ANGEL
OF ETERNAL LIFE
(Use this vision of the beautiful garden
each night as you prepare for sleep.)

Visualize yourself entering a beautiful garden. Colourful flowers and bushes surround you. The sound of birdsong fills the air. Find a white garden bench and sit on it. A beautiful angel, the Angel of Eternal Life, stands there in front of you. He is magnificent, shining with the radiant colours of the sunset. Rays of light stream from his heart centre to yours and the light fills you and renews you. You know that you will visit spiritual realms during your sleep and will wake up refreshed. The angel reminds you that you are a son–daughter of the universe and have your rightful place within it. Everything you do is part of creation, no matter how small it is. You can relax into sleep, knowing that all is well.

Sunday Morning
THE ANGEL OF EARTH

This meditation is intended to renew the strength and vigour of the physical body using the creative powers within it. Think about the things you intend to do during the coming week, or make a 'to-do list' of what you are planning.

BECOME ONE WITH
THE ANGEL OF THE EARTH

Visualize the Angel of the Earth. She is radiant. Her robes of light are shining with all the goodness of the earth. Her colours are the brilliant colours of red, orange and yellow of the summertime and reflect the colours of the grains and fruits of the gardens, fields and trees. As you gaze at her, you see how the seeds and plants of earth grow into edible plants. In the same way, your plans and ideas are nourished and blessed by the Angel of Earth so that they are successful. She will nourish you with new creative thoughts and ideas so that you bring enthusiasm and joy into all you do. Talk to her about the things on your to-do list and receive her encouragement and blessing.

Thursday Evening
The Angel of Wisdom

The power of thought and the ability to think were considered by the Essenes to be cosmic functions as well as a human ability. We see how this concept is being recovered in the twenty-first century by popular films and DVDs, books and films such as 'What the Bleep Do We Know?' and 'The Secret'. Both of these films deal with the 'law of attraction' and how to make it work. The Essenes believed that there was a cosmic ocean of thought that encompassed all the thoughts of the universe and it was a powerful energy. It could never be lost and never reduced. Wisdom brings freedom from fear. It brings peace and perfect health, which are divine gifts.

When preparing for sleep, once again visualize yourself in the beautiful garden of spirit, feeling calm and at one with the Heavenly Father, the Source of All. Sit on a bench and watch the sky, filled with all the colours of the setting sun. The predominant colours are yellow and gold, with flashes of pale orange. These are the colours of spiritual wisdom.

As you admire the colours of the sky, you become aware of the presence of a glorious angel radiating these colours to you. Share with the Angel of Wisdom all the efforts you are making to become a wise and thoughtful person, listening to your inner voice to make the right decisions, guided by infinite and divine intelligence. Ask the Angel of Wisdom to be with you and around you when you need inspiration to make the right decisions. Speak to him about the times your thoughts run away with you, the times when you speak hurtful words that come out like flashes of lightning and cause pain to those you are speaking to. Promise the angel that you will do your best to control your thoughts and words, allowing divine order to manifest in your life.

Friday Morning
THE ANGEL OF AIR

Air is the bridge between matter and spirit. Our lungs are the boundaries between the outside world and us. Not only that, but in many spiritual traditions, the breath is considered holy. This communion was intended to bring attention to the connection between air (breath) and life. We talk about being inspired, and another word for breathing in is inspiration. Breath brings ideas as well as the life-force. The meditation on Friday morning with the Angel of the Air is intended to bring about understanding of the breath as the link between mind and body and the Cosmos, or world of Spirit.

BREATHE IN THE BREATH OF LIFE
A Meditation with the Angel of Air

Welcome the Angel of Air into your life. She inspires your meditations and work. She says:

'Breathe in deeply and fully. Feel energy and vitality enter your body with the breath. Don't struggle or strain. Allow the breath to flow in through your nostrils and down into your lungs. When the lungs are full, relax and the breath will flow out of its own accord. Continue for a few minutes to breathe like this. You can do it outside if there is time and the weather is suitable, or in front of an open window. The air contains invisible life-force that revitalizes you as you breathe like this. You will have more energy and vitality for your daily tasks and will be able to remain calm throughout the day. Continue your breathing and affirm,

'I breathe in life, I breathe out all tension.
I breathe in peace, I breathe out stress.
I breathe in harmony.
The power of life is in my words as I speak
And I am nearer to Mother–Father God.
I am filled with the breath of life.'

Friday Evening
The Heavenly Father

This was the most important communion for the Essenes. As Jews, they began their Sabbath or day of rest at sunset on Friday evening. Today, people welcome Friday as the end of the working week, and even abbreviate 'Thank goodness it's Friday!' to TGIF!

The Essenes dedicated the Friday evening meditation to the Heavenly Father: the Creator, or Source of All–That–Is. It was a special opportunity to concentrate on the universal laws, those that had been dedicated to the Angels of the Earthly Mother and the Heavenly Father during the daily morning and evening meditations. It was also a time to contemplate how human beings fitted harmoniously into the universal scheme of things.

THE EVENING MEDITATION WITH
THE HEAVENLY FATHER

Before sleep, visualize the beautiful Garden of Spirit. You find yourself sitting by the shore of a still lake. The sun is beginning to set, casting a long reflection, like a golden pathway, across the mirror-like surface of the water. All is calm and peaceful. The first stars are beginning to shine. As you prepare to sleep, visualize yourself rising and moving along the pathway of light…. You are entering the kingdom of the Heavenly Father, where you may find peace and tranquillity and spiritual wisdom.

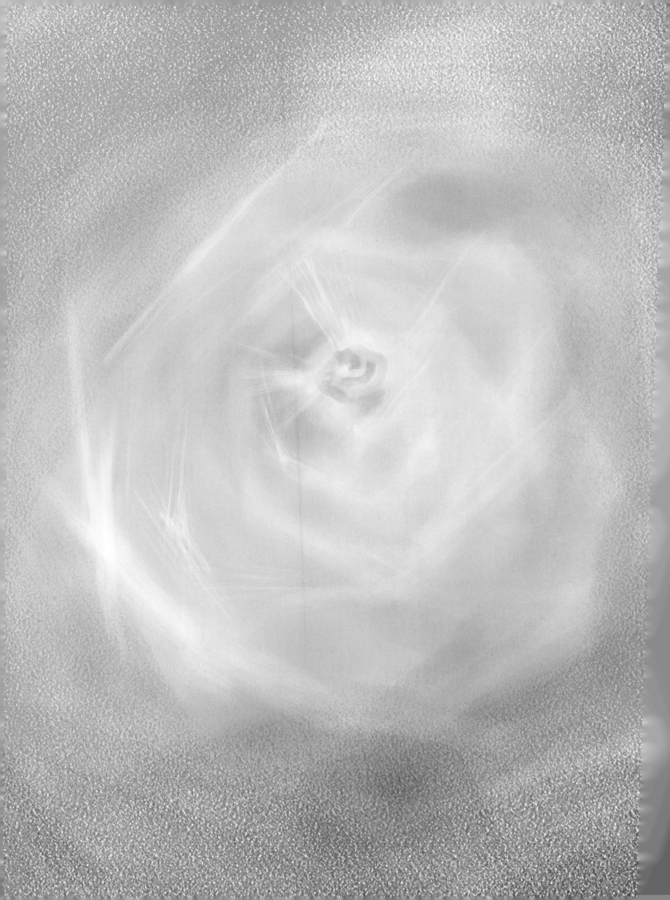

5.
Angels, Colour and the Seven Rays

When you are joyful, your aura is filled with light and colour. Your friends are happy in your company. When you are in a joyful and happy frame of mind, everything you look at seems larger than life. You look at everything through rose-tinted spectacles. Yet life hasn't changed. Your own moods and perceptions are the trigger for this apparent change.

FILL YOUR life with colour. In a moment, we shall discuss the system of the Seven Rays, a way of looking at the spiritual colours of life that goes back to very early times. Each colour of the spectrum corresponds to one of the Seven Rays and brings its qualities and strengths into your life, for colour is very important in our lives. Think how drab everything would be if there were no colours! Colour expresses how we feel and also affects the way we feel. When the sun shines suddenly on a dull and cloudy day, we immediately feel uplifted. Our everyday expressions often refer to our feelings and colour, such as:

In the pink
Green with envy
Got the blues—or
Blue with cold
Red with anger
Yellow with fear

The colours we wear can reflect our feelings or our roles in life. Certain jobs have uniforms that we instantly recognize by their colour, identifying one of the armed forces from another, one supermarket from another, the flight attendants of one airline, or the children of a particular school. Or they may delineate a key worker such as a surgeon from one of their colleagues on the team, such as a nurse. Many uniforms are in serious, sombre colours such as black to convey more authority to the wearer or the company. Wearing particular colours can affect the way we feel. Angels like colour—one of my friends told me emphatically that angels never wear black! Some people have to wear sober or dark colours in their professional life but the aura always shines and reflects its own colour.

There are colours that are connected with your astrological sign. Maybe the colour you choose is important in your horoscope, your sun sign, rising sign or a prominent planet. In her book, *Planetary Harmonies,* the astrologer Joan Hodgson gave the following colours to the sun, moon and planets.

ATTUNEMENT ACTIVITY

Brainstorm a list of any other words or phrases that you associate with feelings and colours.

The Sun rules	Leo	gold or orange
The Moon rules	Cancer	violet or amethyst
Mercury rules	Gemini	pale yellow
and	Virgo	pale orange or corn colour
Venus rules	Taurus	forget-me-not blue or delphinium mauve
and	Libra	gentle blues, shading to green and turquoise
Mars rules	Aries	bright red-orange, scarlet or deep pink
and	Scorpio	rich deep crimson
Jupiter rules	Sagittarius	indigo
and	Pisces	silvery blue-grey
Saturn rules	Capricorn	dark rich green
and	Aquarius	lighter spring green

Some of the spiritual qualities of colours (including the seven colours of the spectrum) are as follows

Red is strength, stability and courage, energy and vitality. It is the colour of our blood, which carries the life-force energy around the body.

Orange is fertility, reproduction, creativity and joy.

Yellow is spiritual wisdom and divine intelligence. It gives the ability to order the thoughts.

Green represents harmony and adaptability. It is the colour of nature, which is cleansing, soothing and healing. It helps us to be non-judgmental and less critical.

Blue is about speaking the truth, for healing and soothing pain. It is a good colour to help with devotion and aspiration.

Indigo helps intuition, inspiration and creative imagination.

Violet represents divine inspiration and spirituality and is another colour of devotion. It is a useful colour to use to enter meditation and connect with your higher self and spirit, with your own guardian or personal angel.

White contains all the colours of the spectrum, and so includes also the spiritual qualities of all the colours. There are also colours which have a slightly different nature from the colours of the spectrum:

Gold is the colour of sunlight, bringing happiness and joy.

Silver is like the moonlight, and is useful for cleansing and protection.

Another colour, pearl, is also used in colour healing systems. It is like a blend of sunlight, moonlight and starlight. It shimmers and shines and its soft sheen of colour is constantly changing. It can also look like mother-of-pearl, found on the inside of shells from which the pearl itself develops. The 'pearl of great price' is a symbol for the most profound spiritual wisdom. In the story, a rich merchant sold everything else he had to buy the most beautiful and precious pearl there had ever been. That pearl represented divine wisdom, like the wisdom of Solomon.

The Seven Rays

By the time the Seven-Ray system had reached the Theosophists in the nineteenth century, a Ray had become a particular name for a type of energy that emphasizes a quality or force and is represented by a colour. They are like beams of light that lead to wisdom. The Seven Rays influence the work you do and your hobbies and interests. There are angels who are the overseers of each type of work, the principalities, who hold the blueprint of its ideal. Principalities are concerned with large organizations, like cities and nations, but also with multinational companies. In spite of all the challenges facing the business world and the workplace, there is an angel who holds the absolute ideal of that work. The people who are devoted and dedicated to the particular employment are inspired by the ideals of the angel. In the same way that the CEO of a company or organization holds its vision, so the over-lighting angel holds the lofty ideal of the business. Employees who are enthusiastic about their tasks can become even more inspired by consciously tuning in to the angel.

We all came to Planet Earth with an ideal to fulfil, but we can forget what that ideal is when we are enmeshed in the different challenges we face. Using colour meditations and the angel of a particular colour or quality provides an opportunity to connect once more with our ideals and begin to enjoy our work life or draw us towards our ideal work.

On the next few pages you will find a brief summary of the Seven-Ray system, the archangels, and the ways they can help us find our ideal mission in life.

THE RED RAY

The First Ray resonates to the colour of red. Its keynote is will, and it inspires people who are active and like to get on and do things. Its spiritual aspect is divine willpower and courage. The ideal work for such people would be as business leaders, like the CEO of a large organization; in the legal system; those who govern, such as MPs and government officers; explorers; soldiers; leaders; drivers of public vehicles, who are responsible for getting passengers safely to their destinations; or surgeons.

The angels for the Red Ray are the angels of willpower, energy and self-confidence. An archangel working with the Red Ray is Archangel Michael. His name means 'He who is like God'.

Affirmation for the Red Ray
I am happy, confident and successful in all I do.

To deepen your connection to the Red Ray, breathe in the perfume of a deep red or crimson damask rose or rose essential oil—or a rhododendron, as below. Use red gemstones like garnets, rubies or red jasper.

A Meditation about Archangel Michael

When you are feeling frustrated or stressed with your work, or want to find inspiration to make changes, it can be helpful to meditate with Archangel Michael. He is often portrayed holding scales of balance. He is also a powerful angel of protection and is often seen with a sword. If you are ever fearful, you can call on him for protection.

ARCHANGEL MICHAEL'S SWORD

For your meditation, play restful music and burn angelica oil or frankincense. As its name suggests, angelica oil is the oil for all angels but particularly Archangel Michael. Sitting in your usual meditation position, begin to centre yourself with your breathing. Feel the cool air at the tip of your nose, and the warm breath as you breath out. Follow the breath into your chest and heart centre and visualize yourself bathed in golden sunlight.

In imagination, begin to rise upwards, as though on a beam of light, and find yourself in a beautiful garden among avenues of fine trees. Looking around, you see a beautiful white building in the distance at the end of one of the vistas. Walk towards it until you find yourself standing in front of it. It is a temple of light. It has an entrance with a finely carved door and there are seven steps of clear quartz leading up to it. You climb the steps, feeling the warmth and smoothness of the crystal under your bare feet. When you reach the double doors, there are handles of gold. Turn the handle and open the door. Inside is a beautiful circular hall. The floor and pillars are clear quartz. The roof is open to the light and it pours in, radiating and sparkling onto the crystal. As it does so, the hall reflects all the colours and shades of the spectrum. Vases with lilies and roses of different shades of red and pink stand around the walls and their scent fills the air. At the centre is a candle, like a pillar, with a still flame burning on it. The candle is level with your heart centre. There are white benches placed around the walls and you sit on one of them.

The atmosphere is peaceful and you feel refreshed and energized. Then you become aware of the presence there of Archangel Michael. He is surrounded with golden light, like the sun. You might see him as a colour or as a vibration, or as he is usually painted in pictures. However you see him or sense him, you know he is there. Archangel Michael is the archangel to call on for removal of energy connected to old memories, events or people and difficulties at work. When you are ready to be released from these old, stuck, situations, Michael uses his sword of light to remove the cords that can tie you to the past.

Ask him now to remove anything that keeps you stuck. Visualize any difficult situations, relationships at home or at work that challenge you, or memories that still haunt you, and then see the sword flashing down all around you as its light cuts these old chords and knots.

Now Michael gives you the sword to hold. It's not heavy. It is weightless, made of pure light. As you hold it, its light fills every part of you. Feel it filling your feet, legs, body, arms, neck and head, as a vase is filled with water. You become filled with light, and it dissolves the shadows of old energy and old memories that you no longer need.

The sword is the sword of truth and justice, and Michael asks you only to use it for the very highest good of all—so that you are able always to work for the light and do your best. You cannot use the sword for anyone else, only yourself. You can always ask Michael to come to you when you need it to remove any stuck situations in your life. Visualize the situation and any chords or threads that seem to stretch from you to it. Then use the sword to cut the chords or ties. Or ask Michael to do it. You give the sword back to Archangel Michael. He takes a candle and lights it from the pillar candle, giving it to you. It is a light to show you the way forward. He asks you what will be the first thing you will do during the coming week that will help you to find the way forward. Tell him any small idea that comes to mind. Big things start with small steps.

Thanking the Archangel, you walk back to the entrance of the temple and down the steps, down the path of light until you find yourself sitting in your own room again. Begin to ground yourself by breathing more deeply, feel the solidity of the floor or the earth beneath you, and start to stretch and open your eyes.

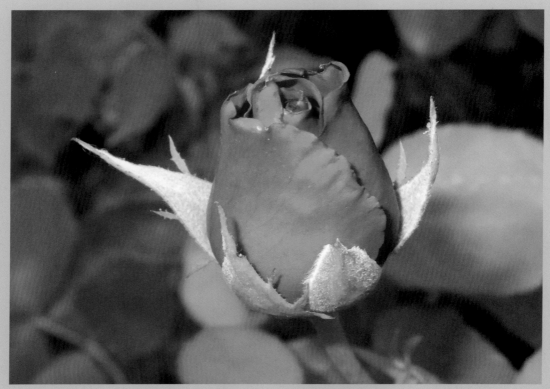

Many years ago, when I was planning an angel workshop, I wanted to do it on Michaelmas Day, Archangel Michael's day, which is September 29th. I did a meditation about it and asked the archangel if the workshop had his blessing. The meditations that follow came to me.

He actually put me through quite a strict test. He asked me what spiritual laws I followed. As a yoga teacher, I follow the guidelines of *Raja Yoga*, which are the first two of the eight limbs of yoga by the sage Patanjali. The first five are practices that are the ethical foundation to live one's life. They are **non-violence, truth, non-stealing, to be sexually faithful or celibate (depending on your circumstances)**, and **absence of greed**. The second five are concerned with personal discipline. They are **purity, contentment, self-discipline, self-study** and **surrender.**

The second group particularly involve letting go and trusting all is well. In the meditation I had a job to remember them all and I had to admit to the archangel I had forgotten one. He told me he had given me a test in honesty, not memory. That was when he gave me the sword to clear old situations that no longer served me. He showed me how to use a spiritual light (candle) to light the way. He showed me how to weigh up a situation with balance scales and a feather (see page 109).

The Orange (Gold) Ray

Visualize a beautiful piece of clear amber with the warmth of the sun shining through it. This helps to understand the Orange Ray, sometimes called Gold.

The keynote of the Second Ray is love. Its spiritual aspect is divine love and it is the Ray of the Divine Mother. The spirit of love and devotion motivates people who are on this ray. It is the ray of teaching and healing, philanthropy, the business world and parents. The Orange Ray inspires teachers who have a real gift for helping youngsters learn. Entrepreneurs who are dedicated to their work and always try to satisfy the needs of their clients show second-ray qualities. People who feel they have a true vocation for the work they do, and do it because they love the work rather than for its financial reward, are strongly influenced by it.

Orange is a stimulating colour and a good one to have by you if you are feeling tired and depleted. Suitable gemstones to hold or wear are clear, bright amber, golden topaz, carnelian or gold tiger-eye. Wearing amber jewellery can help your energy in difficult business meetings that would otherwise leave you drained. You can have a piece in your pocket or briefcase. Gold rings or cufflinks also have an alchemical influence. As well as often being a sign of wealth, they represent the way in which the hard work of our everyday physical life brings spiritual rewards in the mastery of difficulties. Having orange roses in a meeting room also brings in the golden ray energy and the influence of roses can soften the aggression sometimes experienced in meetings.

The angels of the Orange Ray are angels of strength and vitality. An archangel associated with the Orange (Gold) Ray is Archangel Uriel. If your work is associated with the qualities of this ray, you can also visualize an angel of that colour with its qualities.

Affirmations for the Gold Ray:

I am divine wisdom
I am divine strength
I love the work I do and I do the work I love.

Essential oils of orange or mandarin bring the energy of the Orange Ray.

If you want to seek further inspiration about the work you do or want to do, brainstorm a list of ideas and how you might put them into practice. Write three ideas that would enable to you achieve them fairly easily.

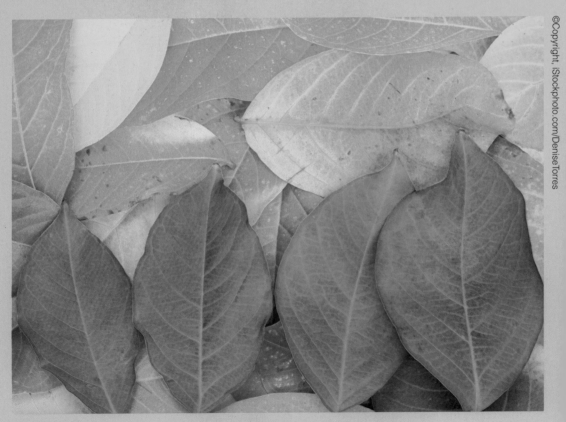

Archangel Uriel's Golden Flame of Strength and Wisdom

Archangel Uriel's name means 'Light of God'. He is often seen with a golden flame in the palm of his hand (see p. 125). Another symbol of Uriel is the lightning flash, representing the planet of Uranus, which is his planet. Visualize Archangel Uriel as an immense golden orange flame surrounding you like a cloak. The flame represents divine love and divine wisdom. Within the flame with you is the archangel, shimmering and shining with flame colours.

A well-known meditation is gazing at a candle flame. (If you suffer from epilepsy or migraines, do this as a visualization only; don't gaze at the actual flame.) Find a candle or tea light and place it in front of you and light it. Draw the curtains so that the room is relatively dark and the flame is bright and clear. Sit in front of the flame, about two feet away. Start to gaze at the candle flame. When your eyes get tired or start to water, close them.

Visualize the flame. It grows larger and larger until it feels as if you are sitting in it. It doesn't burn, it feels pleasantly warm. In the light you see Uriel, a magnificent golden angel. He is like a flame of light and all the colours associated with fire and warmth radiate from him. As you look at him, you feel renewed in energy and filled with strength. If you want to feel more passionate and devoted to the work you do, silently ask Uriel to help you with the flame of strength. Affirm, 'I am divine strength'. If you want to become wiser and more knowing about what you do, affirm 'I am divine wisdom'.

Take some time to visualize the work you do or want to do. Picture the aspects of it that you feel most enthusiastic or passionate about. It is a fact that we need to feel enthusiastic and passionate about our work so that we can do a good job. If you are in a job where you feel frustrated and unhappy, picture any aspect of it that you do enjoy. See it surrounded by the golden flame of strength and energy so you feel keener to give it even more enthusiasm. Thank Archangel Uriel when you are ready to conclude the visualization.

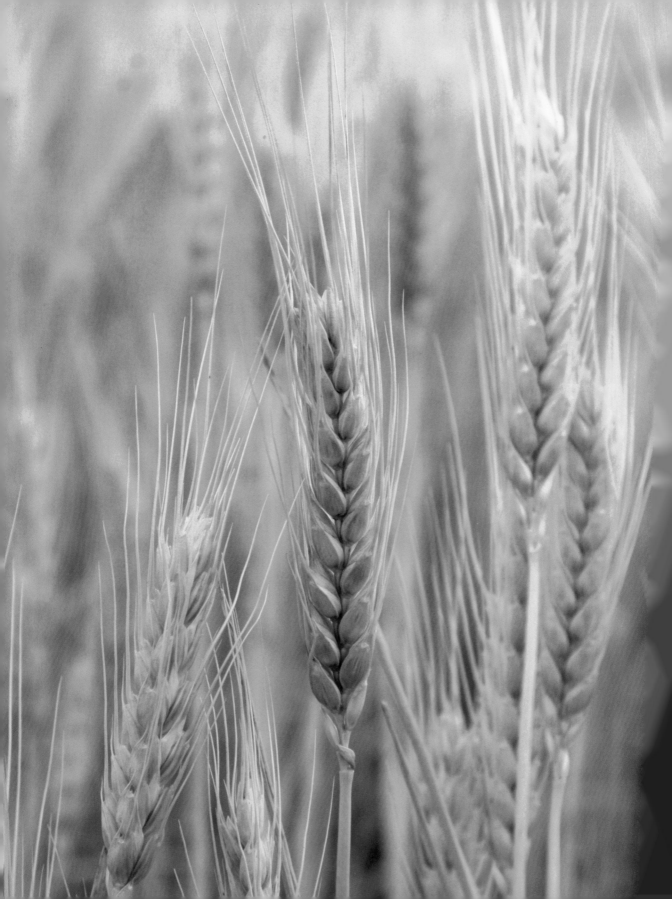

THE YELLOW RAY

Visualizing a beautiful, faceted citrine crystal will bring you into the vibration of the Yellow Ray. Even better is to sit in the sunshine on a beautiful day.

The keynote of the Yellow or Third Ray is communication. The archangel associated with it is Jophiel. His name means 'Beauty of God', and his ray is sometimes called the sunshine ray. It is concerned with wisdom, intelligence and philosophy. It influences writers, journalists, the publishing world and media, people who work on computers and large business organizations. Its spiritual aspect is wisdom and the ability to communicate it successfully. Wisdom is quite different from knowledge. Wisdom brings together knowledge with experience, intuition and inspiration. It is also concerned with adaptability. The person who listens to their inner voice, and business people who follow their hunches and make good decisions, are influenced by the Yellow Ray and the principalities who work with it.

Yellow accessories, ties, yellow flowers in the home or office and yellow gemstones like citrine or rutilated quartz (quartz with enclosures of the mineral rutile, which is generally golden yellow) help the inspiration of this ray. A tiger-eye paperweight on the desk or as an ornament in the office inspires wisdom and communication. Suitable essential oils to use are any of the lemon-scented ones like lemon itself, may chang or lemongrass, or grapefruit. Using them in an electric vaporizer or oil burner immediately lifts the spirits and refreshes the atmosphere, enabling clarity of thought.

The angels of the Yellow Ray are angels of spiritual wisdom. The gold of spiritual wisdom is recognized in art, where Jesus Christ, angels, gurus, gods and saints are all depicted with a golden halo.

Affirmations for the Yellow Ray:
I am divine wisdom
I am inspired by my spiritual wisdom
I am flexible and adaptable and I shall always
make the right decision.

Yellow Roses Meditation

Roses are generally acknowledged to be beautiful flowers and yellow ones bring the energy of beauty and wisdom. As the rose pours forth its perfume, it inspires everyone with happiness and joy. If you have a yellow rose, place it in front of you, or else use a picture. (Greetings cards often have beautiful photographs of flowers or other suitable scenes to inspire meditation.)

Use essential oil of rose in the oil burner, for devotion to the yellow ray. Use lemon, grapefruit or may chang for mental clarity. Spend some time looking at the rose and imprinting its image in your mind.

Then close your eyes and become aware of each breath. Follow the breath into your chest and into the heart chakra at the centre. Visualize there a perfect rose. Imagine the delicate perfume. Feel the soft silky petals, as though you are in the rose. The petals are opening in the sunlight. Every petal seems to shine and sparkle with light.

At the centre of the rose there shines a sparkling drop of dew. As the light shines on it, it radiates all the colours of the spectrum, as a diamond does. You feel as if you yourself are becoming light. Every atom and cell shines and sparkles with light. Within the diamond dewdrop you see every colour of the spectrum.

Each colour has a quality and they represent all the qualities within you that you have developed through all your experiences. Each challenge and opportunity you have dealt with has inspired a quality of strength and wisdom that are shown in the colours of your diamond in your heart chakra. The famous Buddhist mantra, 'Om Mani Padme Hum', means 'the jewel of enlightenment shines in my heart's lotus'. This drop of diamond-like dew represents the lotus of enlightenment and wisdom.

Archangel Jophiel stands before you and reminds you that you are a strong and wise person, who has gained wisdom from all of life's experiences. Tell Jophiel of any experience that has helped you find strength, courage and wisdom that you are proud of. He reminds you that the work you do is an important contribution to your family, your community or to society as a whole. At any time you can ask the principality concerned to help you to do your best to fulfil the ideal of the work you do. Spend some time remembering why you chose to do your work. It could have chosen you, of course. All work, including caring for relatives at home, is honourable and the angel concerned will give you strength to do your best even at challenging times.

Conclude your meditation when you are finished, in the way given (p. 27).

The Green Ray

Imagine a beautiful cut emerald of high quality. As the sun shines on it and through it, all the other colours of the spectrum are seen with its green tones.

The keynotes of the Green Ray, which is the Fourth of the Rays, are beauty, harmony, balance and peace. It is also concerned with health and healing. It influences artists and designers and healers. Artists and designers attempt to bring the beauty of the higher spiritual world and dimensions into the third dimension. People who are in tune with the Green Ray particularly enjoy being out in the country or in a beautiful park or garden, where the beauty of nature and soothing shades of green surrounds them. Suitable gemstones for helping to find the energy of this ray are emeralds, green calcite, malachite and chrysocolla. Moldavite, a kind of green meteorite glass, which crystallized as it fell to earth from outer space, helps the connection with the angelic kingdom.

Eucalyptus trees are particularly associated with the Green Ray. Their heart-shaped leaves resonate with the heart chakra and the green ray and the essential oil from its leaves helps us to breathe easily and open the heart.

The angels for the Green Ray are those of the keynotes, and also abundance.

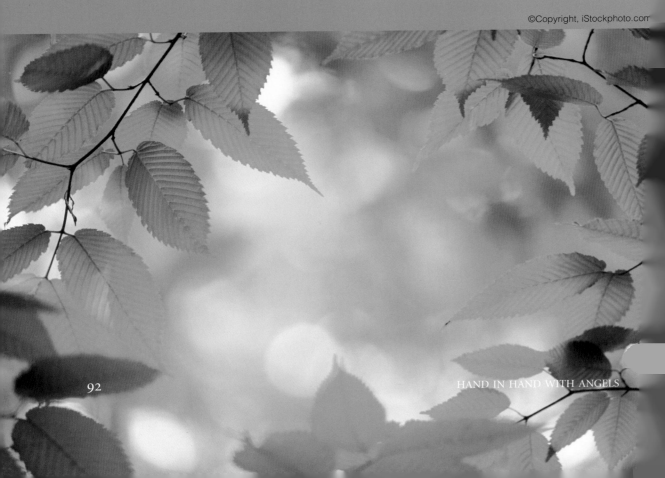

The Temple in the Forest

Centre yourself by tuning in to your breathing and feel yourself growing peaceful and calm. Visualize the sun shining above your head. As you breathe, rays of light begin to surround you until you feel that you are sitting in a canopy of sunlight. Warm rays of light fill your whole being as you breathe and you feel that you are travelling upwards on a path of light, until you find yourself in a beautiful forest glade. Mighty trees surround you. There are fir trees as well as other woodland trees like oak, beech and sycamore. The glade is a clearing like a great circle filled with soft green grass and wild flowers of many colours bloom in it. On each side of the circle you see a path leading into the clearing. You are standing on one of the paths and there is one at the centre of the circle on your right, one to the left, and another ahead of you on the opposite side of the circle. It is like a natural 'medicine wheel' or sacred circle with a path at each of the directions—east, south, west and north.

Walk into the circle, feeling the softness of the grass beneath your feet. Smell the delicate scent of the wild flowers. The sun is warm, and refreshing breezes bring fragrant scents of trees, shrubs and flowers. There are brightly coloured butterflies, and you can hear the hum of other insects and the songs of woodland birds.

When you reach the centre of the clearing, there is a beautiful spring of clear water that bubbles up between rocks and stones in the ground. It spreads out to form a shallow pool with a clear sandy floor. You stoop down, cupping your hands to drink the cool, refreshing water. It tastes so fresh and sweet that it is like the elixir of life. As you splash your face and head and bathe your feet you begin to feel totally alive and invigorated. Looking at the sandy floor of the pool, you see something shining in it. It is a beautiful coloured pebble, worn smooth by the water that constantly bubbles into the pool from the spring. You bend down to pick it up, examining its colour, texture and markings. It is a green gemstone that has been waiting for you to come and find it. Its surface has been polished by the ages of time that it has spent lying in the bubbling spring waiting for you. Its special gift for you is to bring more inspiration and creativity into your life and work. Sit by the pool enjoying the warmth of the sun.

Now you feel that someone is coming towards you. It is a beautiful angel, Archangel Raphael, the archangel of abundance. You recognize him and are pleased to see him. He sits beside you and you are able to ask his advice about improving your work life, applying for promotion, changing jobs or finding more congenial work. Discuss with him any issues you wish to. You may hear

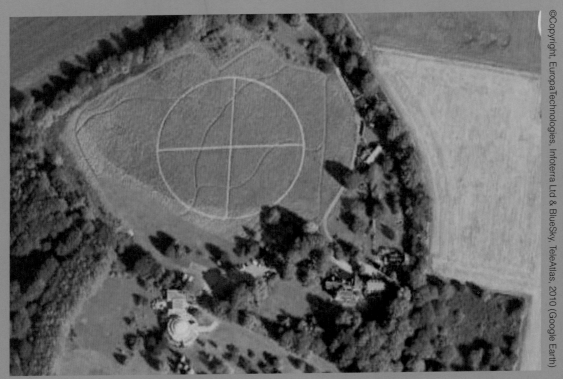

advice or see symbols, pictures or get ideas. Be ready to consider any likely possibilities.

It is time to return to your everyday awareness. Thank Raphael and turn to go back across the clearing and along the path, travelling down the pathway of light back into your everyday self. Begin to breathe more deeply and open your eyes when you are ready. Take some time to feel sure that you are grounded into everyday consciousness once again.

Affirmations for the Green Ray:

I am always inspired by my creative ability
I am open to divine inspiration.

When I experienced for myself the meditation in the previous page, I didn't realize that some time after there would be a beautiful mown grass 'medicine wheel' or circle with a path at each of the four directions at New Lands, country home of the White Eagle Lodge. You can see it in the photo; the alignment of the compass points is exact, although slightly distorted by the angle at which the picture was taken.

HAND IN HAND WITH ANGELS

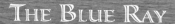

THE BLUE RAY

Visualize a brilliant sapphire. It is very clear and translucent and cut in such a way that the light refracts all the colours of the spectrum through its vivid blueness.

This Fifth Ray resonates with scientists and all who seek diligently in the search for truth and knowledge. It is another ray of wisdom. Its keynote is concrete knowledge and analytical science. The Blue Ray influences scientists and researchers who devote everything to scientific discovery, such as Marie Curie. It is also the ray of those who search for spiritual truth, like saints and gurus of all ages and those who seek secrets of healing to benefit all. Creative artists, who attempt to bring beauty and harmony to enhance the quality of life, are also influenced by it. The spiritual aspect of the Blue Ray and its angels are creativity, balance, justice, truth, peace and protection.

As well as sapphires, other suitable gemstones are kyanite, blue lace agate, aquamarine, larimar and the two special angel stones, angelite and celestite. Blue flowers like forget-me-nots and bluebells, along with shrubs like blue hydrangeas, also resonate with the Blue Ray. I always think of a bluebell wood when I visualize the blue ray, or the brilliant blue sky of lazy summer days. If you have the chance to visit a bluebell wood at the height of the season (April and May), just walking through the woods and inhaling the scent of the flowers will assist attunement to the Blue Ray. Or remember sitting by the sea and looking out towards the horizon, seeing shades of blue of the sea and sky stretching into the distance!

Affirmations for the Blue Ray:
I always listen to my inner wisdom and truth
I rely on truthful guidance to make the right decisions
I am at peace

The Healing Pool and Archangel Gabriel

To enhance this meditation, have blue flowers or a blue candle in front of you and hold a blue gemstone. Celestite is a good one to hold or have in front of you, as it is an angelic messenger. It helps to make a clear connection to the angels, as its name suggests. It is celestial, like the blue of the sky. It is a good stone to bring your acceptance that angels are really with you and that you have a God-given right to communicate with them. Celestite is a stone of truth and wisdom and helps to bring awareness of the highest state of truth. If something is worrying you in your working life this is a particularly cleansing meditation to do. It will tend to wash away the confusion so that you can make clear decisions. Archangel Gabriel is the celestial messenger and using celestite makes a deeper connection with him. Gabriel means 'God is my Strength' or 'Power of God'.

You are sitting in a beautiful garden beside a peaceful still pool. The sun is shining and the blue sky is reflected in the surface of the water, which is like a mirror. Around you are blue flowers and shrubs. The pool has steps and a paved border, both of blue stones that glisten in the sunlight. Go and sit on the steps by its edge. Dip your feet in the pure, clear water. The water is cool and refreshing and you decide to bathe in it. You can swim or float or paddle, whatever suits you. You begin to feel really cleansed and refreshed, and reinvigorated. The water is so clear that you can see right to the bottom of the pool, which is paved with the same smooth blue stones. In the same way that the water is clear and reflects the blue sky, so you are able to reflect the clarity and guidance of your higher self.

When you come out of the pool, you see a magnificent angel waiting for you. The angel is wearing a cloak of all shades of clear blue, the shades of the sky and the sea, shot through with pure light and glimpses of gold, like the sun. His robe is like pure light. It is Archangel Gabriel, who works for truth, peace and purity. He is waiting for you and has a special gift for you.

As you step out of the water and up the steps, you feel pure and light again. Gabriel places a blue cloak around your shoulders. He tells you that whenever you need to understand a situation and know what to do, you can visualize yourself in the blue cloak and it will help things to become clear. When you have work decisions to consider, visualize yourself in the blue cloak. It will help you to become more creative and imaginative in the work you do.

The Indigo Ray

Think of beautiful dark blue gemstones like azurite, iolite, sodalite and lapis lazuli. The Sixth or Indigo Ray is the ray of devotion and religious aspiration. It is the ray of the true mystic and those who are devoted to their religion or to a saint or guru. People influenced by this ray are very idealistic, and it is another ray of love. The angels of this ray are the angels of love and wisdom. The Archangel appropriate to it is Raziel. His name means 'Secret of God' or 'Angel of Mysteries'. Ancient stories say that he gave his Book of Wisdom to Adam. It was later passed to the prophet Enoch. Apparently, only wise people devoted to truth and immune from corruption would be able to understand the book. Later the Book of Wisdom was given to Noah to help him to build the ark. It was passed down until it came to King Solomon, famed for the wisdom he learned from it. It is said that anyone who has a sudden revelation, an 'aha' moment, is tuned in to Raziel and the Book of Wisdom. Raziel's guidance is very concerned with lateral thinking, not orthodox means. According to the angel author, Theolyn Cortens, working with Raziel is likely to bring sudden changes in to your life.*

Working with Archangels

Affirmations for the Indigo Ray:

I see with spiritual vision
I am divine wisdom
Aum
(the ancient Sanskrit word used frequently as a mantra)

I acknowledge my own intuition and power to know, which now manifests in my life in perfect and harmonious ways, under grace and in divine right order.

I like to use iolite with the Indigo Ray. In the vision quests of the Native Americans and Shamans, it is a guide or prophecy stone. It acts as a guardian when you go on inner or outer journeys of self-exploration. It awakens inner wisdom and clears confusion about your life purpose. Iolite is a rare stone, available only from specialist shops.

The Vision Quest

This meditation is like a vision quest. It is a special one to do when you feel at a crossroads in life. In traditional communities, a vision quest is often done when setting out anew in life or at special times or when making important decisions.

Hold an iolite crystal or wear an item of iolite jewellery. Tune in to your breathing. Notice each breath as it comes and goes. Then direct each breath into the crystal. Visualize yourself standing outside a magnificent building, which is a library. It has a beautiful door and steps leading up to it. You walk in to the library and find yourself in a reception hall. The floor is decorated with a pattern of tiles and there is a large staircase ahead of you. Walk up the stairs and you find yourself in a long corridor with doors on each side. Each door has a name in letters of gold but you know you can only read the door with your own name on it. When you find that door, walk into the room. It holds all the records of your life. There are shelves around the room and the books are all about the wonderful things you have done. Remember, there are no mistakes, because you will have learned something from the things you thought were wrong. In the middle of the room, there is a large wooden table. It is round and has carved legs. There are carved, polished chairs around the table. On the table is a beautiful book. Use your creative imagination to design the book and its cover. Maybe it is leather or other material like silk or velvet, covered with fine lettering or gemstones. It is the most beautiful book you can imagine. It is your Book of Wisdom, which holds the records of your life and life purpose.

Ask Archangel Raziel to be with you. He is usually shown carrying the Book of Wisdom. Ask him to show you your true self, beyond the outer personality. You may ask to be reminded of your life purpose or how to make positive changes in your life. Raziel goes to the table and you both sit at it. He opens your Book of Wisdom at the page you have reached in your life. He shows you it. Look at the page and read what is there. It may appear in pictures or symbols or insights may come to you later in lucid dreams or at another time. Be confident that whatever you wish to know or do will happen in some way. Raziel may say something to you, which you hear mentally or see as a symbol.

Thank Raziel and leave the library the way you came in. Finish your meditation in the usual way.

THE VIOLET OR
AMETHYST RAY

Think of beautiful amethysts, their hue reaching from palest lilac to deepest violet. The amethyst is a calming and protective stone that aids the deepest meditation. Think also of ametrine, the beautiful stone that combines both amethyst and citrine; of charoite and sugelite, both deep purple gemstones that open the crown chakra to spiritual inspiration.

The Amethyst Ray, the Seventh Ray, is a ray of transformation and alchemy, the meeting place of spirit and matter. In the chakra system, it represents the crown chakra, the place of spiritual inspiration. It is the ray of divine love, divine order and of ceremony, which includes not only religious ceremony but also ceremonies of state. Think of national ceremonies of all kinds, such as the inauguration of a president, a coronation, weddings, state funerals, and the Olympic Games with its ceremony of lighting and carrying the Olympic flame and the ceremony of presenting the medals. Every event, from the smallest personal or family one to civic, national or international events, call on the highest ideals that ceremony can represent. It is also the ray of the Violet Flame of Transformation.

Theatre and drama come under the influence of the Violet Ray, as do true psychics and mystics and students of the Inner Mysteries or Ancient Wisdom. Alchemists, who work to transmute base metal—the physical body—into the pure gold of spirit are associated with the Violet ray.

The angel of the Violet Ray is Archangel Zadkiel. His name means 'Righteousness of God' and he is the angel of mercy and benevolence. He prevented Abraham from sacrificing his son Isaac. He enhances the meditative experience, bringing spiritual inspiration, and works on the Violet Ray to cleanse and protect. Zadkiel teaches the use of the violet flame meditation to assist people to release old trauma and negative and destructive habits.

The Violet Ray is the ray of the new Age of Aquarius, the age of brotherhood and unity, of co-operation. It is a very subtle ray and is closely associated with higher levels of meditation like *Samadhi, Nirvana* and Enlightenment. The story of the Sorcerer's Apprentice tells us what happens when someone tries to use psychic powers before they are ready.

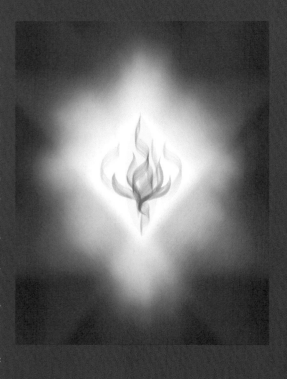

Affirmations for the Violet Ray:

Divine order is now established in my
personal and business affairs.
I am one with the Light, the source of
All That Is, the Creator.
I am pure and light.

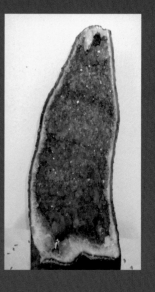

To enhance meditation on the the Seventh Ray, use violets, lilac or any purple or lilac-coloured flowers in season. Wear amethyst jewellery, or amethyst scarf or t-shirt if you have any of these. Suitable essential oils are frankincense, jasmine or neroli.

The Violet Flame

As you enter into a deep state of meditation, you become aware that you are standing on a pavement of the deepest shade of amethyst. The stones are formed of pure amethyst crystal. They feel warm under your feet. As you look around, you see that you are standing on a processional way, a track that stretches far ahead. There are tall columns on each side, also formed of amethyst. Ahead of you is a beautiful circular amethyst temple. You enter the temple through an arched doorway and inside there are benches arranged in a circle. At the centre is an amethyst altar shaped like a double cube with a simple flame burning on the top.

Sit on one of the benches and invite your personal angel to sit with you. As it does so, the Archangel Zadkiel also comes. Use your creative imagination to see what he looks like.

Zadkiel helps you to use the violet flame of cleansing and healing to transmute any negative traits you have. You see that the flame on the altar burns in all shades of deepest violet to palest lilac, white and silver. Zadkiel stands before you and begins to radiate the same colours as the altar flame. You become bathed in shades of violet and silver. You are filled and surrounded by the violet flame. It reaches from beneath your feet to above your head and surrounds you on all sides. It moves and flickers like living flame, filling every atom and cell of your whole being with its light. It has the ability to transmute all negativity in you. If you want to give up smoking and drinking, eating too much, bad temper or impatience, visualize the violet flame dissolving them. See it flickering and rubbing all over you. It rises up around and through your body from your feet to the crown of your head and radiates out around you like a fountain of living liquid light and flame. Repeat the affirmation, 'I am pure and light. All is in Divine Order in my personal and business affairs as I do my perfect work'.

When you are ready, the violet flame fades away and the light on the central altar begins to shine out like a beacon of light to transmute all negativity from Planet Earth.

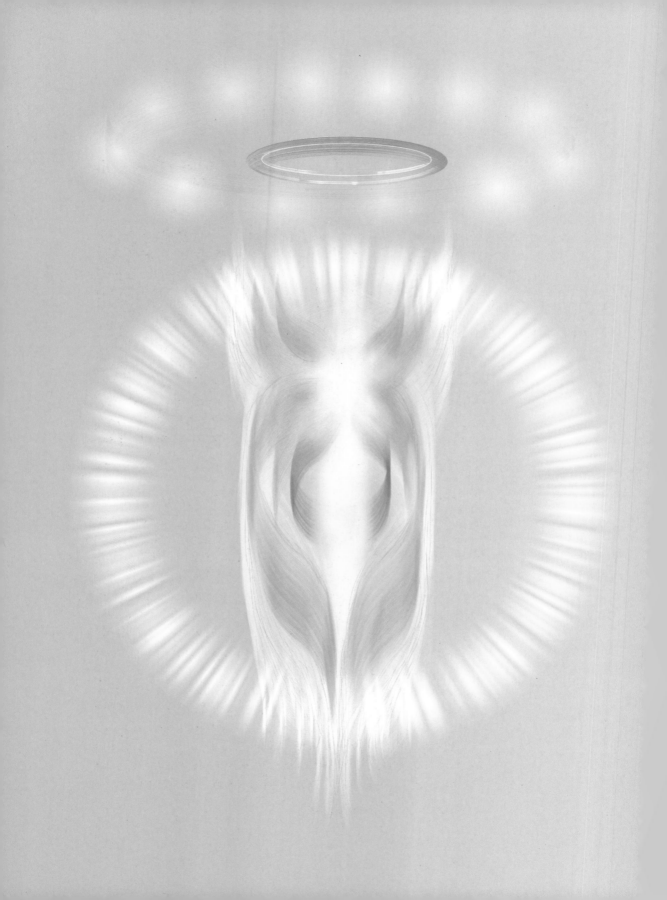

6.

Four Archangels

Find that place of stillness within you where we can communicate with you. It is infinite space, as deep and infinite as the space in the heavens that scientists investigate and explore, discovering more and more as the years go by. It is the same with the infinite space within you. It is unfathomable until you begin to travel into it. Each time you enter into the infinity that is within you, the greater the vista that reveals itself. A whole universe can be found within your own DNA. Its spiral reflects the nebulae and galaxies. It is written, 'As above, so below'. Find that secret place within, in meditation, and as you meditate daily, so you become *as one* and you become whole … holy.

THERE IS often confusion about the role of archangels, who are mentioned as only in the second ranking above angels themselves. After all, Michael's name means 'He who is as God', and he is reputed to have won the battle against Satan in a heavenly war between good and evil. He is mentioned as a prince of the Seraphim, the highest rank of the ascending hierarchy. We tend to use 'archangel' as a generic term for anything higher than an angel—although there's maybe the point that angels are actually unclassifiable!

Archangels are the messengers of God. Apart from guardian angels, they are the ones best known by people and most often seen. In most Christian writing, only two archangels are generally referred to: Gabriel and Michael. But the other traditions that give importance to angels, such as Zoroastrianism, mention at least four, adding Raphael and

Uriel to these two. That makes four archangels whose names are well known: Raphael, Michael, Gabriel and Uriel (also spelt Auriel or Oriel). They often represent the four elements, fire, earth, air and water.

In the Native American tradition, the elements also link with the points of the compass, in the medicine wheel. Today we tend to say 'north, south, east, west' and, following the clock face, we start the cycle at north. The medicine wheel does not begin with the north; instead it begins with the east, the place of the sunrise, the dawn. The east is the place of new beginnings, of enlightenment. In the Annual Calendar it is when the sun is in Aries, the time of spring and the New Year. The New Year of January 1st is a man-made calendar. The real New Year in the astrological sense is when the sun moves into Aries on or about March 21st, the spring equinox (in the northern hemisphere—readers in the southern hemisphere will have to adapt what I say!). The New Year then corresponds to the dawn in the daily cycle. It is a time of new beginnings. Some spiritual traditions face the east, the dawn and time of new light, for their prayer and meditation, as it is a place of enlightenment.

Raphael is traditionally the archangel of the east. He represents the element of air. Certainly, in the northern hemisphere we experience March winds (air) and often wild weather at the time of the equinox. The archangel of the south is Michael, representing the warmth of the sun and the element of fire. The time of day that matches south is noon and the time of year is the summer solstice, when the sun enters the zodiacal sign of Gemini on or about June 21st. Gabriel is the archangel of the west and the element of water. The time of day he represents is the evening and the time of year is the autumn equinox, about September 21st, when the sun enters Libra. Uriel (Auriel) is the archangel of the north, of the element of earth and the winter solstice, which falls around December 21st, when the sun enters Capricorn.

Archangel Gabriel

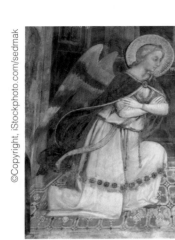

Gabriel kneels before Mary in this detail of a fresco in the church of San Miniato al Monte, Florence, Italy

Probably the best known of the four is Archangel Gabriel. He appeared to Mary to tell her that she would give birth to Jesus. As Jibril, the Angel of Truth, he is said to have dictated the holy book, the Koran, to Mohammed. Sometimes Gabriel is depicted as feminine.

Gabriel doesn't always show him- or herself clearly in meditation or visions but can be mysterious, by calling your attention in small ways. Recently, I did a one-day workshop about him. It was to be in February and I announced it at the end of the previous November. During the month of December, there were over four hundred hits on a meditation about Gabriel that I had written for our website. It remains high on the list of popularity of our website meditations. Whenever I switched on the radio, it seemed to be playing the music 'Gabriel's Oboe'. Then a friend, Ron, painted a picture of white lilies, Gabriel's flower, for me for a Christmas present. When I went to the supermarket to buy flowers for the workshop, there was one bunch of trumpet lilies, the kind seen with Gabriel in pictures. I had never noticed that kind of lily in the supermarket before. Then another friend, Jo, gave me a fridge magnet of Gabriel, which I actually put on my computer for inspiration in writing.

Gabriel is well known as a heavenly messenger. Because he announced the coming of Jesus to Mother Mary, and the birth of John the Baptist to Elizabeth, he is associated with fertility, creativity and change, and new beginnings. As the inspirer of the Koran, he is also associated with communication and writing, and with truth and purity. These are all aspects of our everyday work that we can ask Gabriel to help with.

The meditation on Gabriel overleaf is helpful if you want to make positive changes in your life. Prepare for it by making the three lists, as set out in the Attunement Activity alongside the meditation.

Archangel Gabriel and the White Lily Initiation

For this meditation, use incense or essential oil in a burner to help to make a strong connection with Gabriel. Frankincense, sandalwood and myrrh are good oils for this meditation. Celestite or rutilated quartz are both helpful crystals to use to deepen the connection. Burn a white candle for pure intention. Feel the firmness of the ground, of Mother Earth, beneath you. You feel safe and know that Mother Earth supports you on your inner journey to visit Archangel Gabriel.

Begin to breathe deeply and slowly. With your mind's eye, your inner vision, see yourself surrounded by a sphere of white, sparkling, shimmering light. Within the light you see a beautiful angelic being. It is the Archangel Gabriel, God's messenger. Gabriel is in translucent sparkling white robes, yet you can also see all of the colours of the rainbow scintillating and radiating within the whiteness, like a diamond that shines and glitters in the sunlight. Gabriel's aura is like the purest gold, looking like wings surrounding him. As you look into Gabriel's eyes you feel truly loved. He gives you an affirmation.

I AM always loved and filled with love.

Gabriel takes you by the hand and you go into a beautiful garden. You see magnificent roses of all colours. There are seats in the rose garden and you sit on one with the archangel. Gabriel reminds you that the lists that you made mean you have given away all your worries to God and the angels. Affirm,

I AM filled with God's loving energy and strength.

You walk through the garden with Gabriel until you come to a beautiful bed of white lilies. The air is filled

ATTUNEMENT ACTIVITY

The first list (see p. 105) can be headed 'money and worries'. Write any of your current concerns about these on the list. Make another list headed 'relationships'. Write any concerns about relationships with friends, family or colleagues here. Make a third list of any worries you have about health matters. After you have finished, if you have the facilities to burn the lists, tear them up into little pieces and burn them in a safe place. If you can't do that, you can flush them away. This helps you to clear away old worries and fears that hold you back from making positive changes.

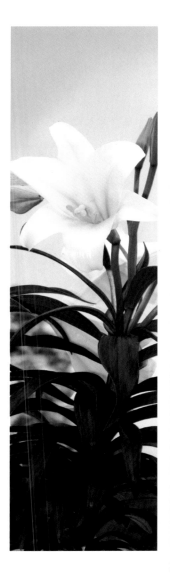

with their beautiful perfume. As you sit by the bed of lilies, the archangel comes close and gazes lovingly into your eyes. His beautiful face is opposite yours and his beautiful blue violet eyes are full of love for you. He gives you another affirmation:

All I do is done with love.

Gabriel turns to the lilies and picks a beautiful lily, which he puts into your hands. He is able to look deep into your heart and see innocence, purity and devotion, for angels see us as we were first created and as we truly are. The lily is a symbol of your birth into a time when you may do the highest work you are able to do and fulfil your greatest potential. It is 'the initiation of the white lily'.

As you hold this beautiful flower, you feel strengthened and renewed and able to face your life with love and gratitude. You can use this beautiful lily in your meditations to help you make right decisions. Visualize yourself holding it. Think of a project you are planning. Look at the lily. Is it beautiful and shining? Or has it faded? If you feel that the lily has faded, check it is not just your fears distorting the image, but if not maybe there is something you need to look at in your project. What would revitalize it? Gabriel gives you a final affirmation:

I am always happy, confident, loving
and successful in all I do.

Now Gabriel takes you by the hand and brings you back into your sphere of light. Sitting in your room, once again you feel the firmness and support of Mother Earth. You breathe slowly and deeply, bringing your mind back to the present. Start to stretch, rub your hands together to generate warmth and cup them over your closed eyes. Feel the warmth in your eyes as you slowly open them. and gently massage your face. Have a good stretch and drink some water to ground yourself.

Archangel Michael

In the Old Testament, Michael is described as one of the strongest guardian angels and as the guardian angel of Israel (Daniel 10). Traditionally, it is said that Satan trembles at the very mention of his name. Michael is often seen in art as trampling a dragon or serpent underfoot.

The dragon or serpent symbolizes our dark side. Michael is a champion of the weak and a great enemy of evil. He represents the triumph of Divine Order over darkness. A Moslem legend speaks of the cherubim being formed from Michael's tears as he weeps over the sins of the faithful.

In Europe and the British Isles there are many churches dedicated to Michael, usually on hilltops. Two of the most famous are St Michael's Mount, in Mount's Bay, near Penzance in Cornwall, and Mont St Michel in Normandy, France. These are both high mounds of rock and vegetation, with a shrine on the top, that rise out of the sea and are only accessible by boat or causeway. At low tide, the causeway is exposed and people can walk across.

According to local legends, Michael appeared to fishermen off the island in Cornwall in 495 AD, and in 708 AD to St Aubert, Bishop of Avranches in France. A similar mount, or mound, is known as Glastonbury Tor. Although not now surrounded by water, it is set in the Somerset Levels, a low-lying area once thought to have been under water. On the top of the Tor is a ruined tower that was part of a church dedicated to Michael.

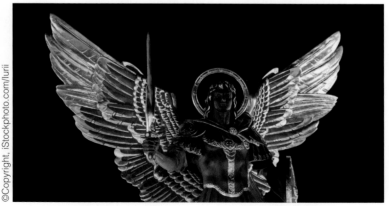

A statue of Archangel Michael, at Maydan Nezalejnosti, Kiev, Ukraine

HAND IN HAND WITH ANGELS

This meditation
is intended to
help you make a
particular decision.
Write down your
ideas in your
meditation journal
so that you fully
remember the
nature of your
inspiration and
where it seems to
point.

Meditation on Archangel Michael

Meditation on Archangel Michael is helpful when you are undecided about the right action to take in any situation.

Make yourself comfortable and begin to centre yourself with your breath. Notice every breath as you breathe in and out. See it as light and spiritual energy from the Source of All-That-Is. It flows down through the crown of the head, filling your body with radiant, sparkling light. You are protected and uplifted by this spiritual light.

Within the light, you see the magnificent form of Archangel Michael. Michael has a gift for you. When you are undecided about what to do, visualize yourself holding a set of balance scales. On one scale is a white feather. On the other scale, visualize a picture or symbol of the issue that concerns you. Picture the choice you need to make. If the scale with the feather rises up, consider your options carefully, as your decision might not be in your best interests. If the scale with your choice rises up, it is the right choice for you.

You can do this with several images of the situation, according to the different possibilities that face you. When you have decided on the right action to take, conclude your meditation by thanking the archangel. Take three deeper breaths and feel your connection to the earth. Become connected again with your everyday self.

Archangel Raphael

We have already discovered quite a lot about Raphael in chapter three, 'Angels and Healing', where there is an Archangel Raphael attunement meditation (pp. 54–5). The traditional stories about the archangel give clues to as to what type of things they help people with. In the story of Tobias, we saw how he healed Sarah and Tobit. The other clues in the story of Tobias are the protection Raphael provided to him on the journey and from the demon. He also collected the money that was owing to Tobit when he really needed it. Raphael helps travellers with protection and abundance to the righteous people who work hard but have difficulties in making ends meet. He is the archangel of travel and safety. When you have to make journeys, you can call Archangel Raphael to help and protect you.

Raphael is included among the seven angels before God mentioned in the Book of Revelation in the New Testament. He also belongs to four of the orders of angels—seraphim, cherubim, dominions and powers. He is the angel of prayer, peace, joy, light and love. Raphael is charged with healing the earth and is also the guardian of the Tree of Life in the Garden of Eden. The gifts of Raphael include knowledge of healing herbs and plants, and healing with colour.

Archangel Uriel

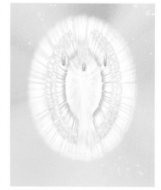

Perhaps Uriel (Auriel) is the least known of the four archangels who have special care for humanity. He is another of the seven angels before the throne of God. He keeps the law of order and harmony and he is a great harmonizer and balancer. He confronts people who have lost their way spiritually to help them find themselves and their purpose in life. Uriel is often known as the Angel of Repentance and helps people to face up to life's difficulties and overcome them. He brings stability and strength to difficulties and challenges.

Uriel is also the Angel of Music and Poetry. Four hundred years ago and more, the poet John Milton gave him quite a big part to play in *Paradise Lost* and called him 'Regent of the Sun'. He is outwitted for a while by Satan, who is the 'he' when this passage begins:

> 'He drew not nigh unheard; the Angel bright,
> Ere he drew nigh, his radiant visage turned,
> Admonished by his ear, and straight was known
> The Arch-Angel Uriel, one of the seven
> Who in God's presence, nearest to his throne,
> Stand ready at command, and are his eyes
> That run through all the Heavens, or down to the Earth
> Bear his swift errands over moist and dry,
> O'er sea and land.'

Many writers and composers talk about the muse who inspires them. The famous eighteenth-century composer, Josef Haydn, basing his story on Milton, included him in his oratorio *The Creation*.

Haydn always wore a ring on his little finger and said he couldn't compose and conduct if he wasn't wearing it. Perhaps it was a link with Uriel that inspired him, because Haydn composed over a hundred symphonies and other famous works! Uriel is particularly associated with the power of thought and the realm of ideas, creativity, insights and judgment, teaching people how to create by using positive thought. He inspires authors who write about affirmations, and may be behind the many books now available about creating healing through visualization and meditation, as well as popular self-help books that encourage people to create what they need in their lives.

Uriel brings a specific link to spiritual realms and shows people how to find their inner power that will help them to reach a higher level of consciousness. We saw earlier how Uriel is the keeper of the golden flame and is often seen with a flame in the palm of his hand. This is a symbol of the spiritual fire known as *kundalini*, which is stored at the base of the spine waiting to be awoken by spiritual means, such as meditation, yoga and ethical living.

Once I had a connection with Haydn, in an unusual way. In August 1991 I had applied for early retirement. I had the chance to stay with a friend at the Order of the Cross at their centre, which was then in Newbury. She taught natural movement and dance and they were going to dance or sing Haydn's *Creation*. You could choose which medium you wanted. I wanted to create the work I now do! In the end I decided to dance it, but I also went to the singing practices. While I was there, I also wrote a poem, which is in my meditation notebook to this day. That week was also a tremendous relief to me from studying for my MA, which took four years when I was also doing a full-time job. This is the poem I wrote then.

Beloved Father–Mother of all life
Of all Creation
Who was present at my birth
And at all my difficulties
Pour out the light of your grace
On me
So
That every atom and cell
Of my being
May be created anew
And I radiate light
Wherever I go

These four archangels are particularly associated with Planet Earth and have spent aeons of time working with the human race to make the planet a safe and beautiful place to live. They are always willing to work with people who have the best interests of the planet and its inhabitants at heart. Be confident that you can contact these powerful archangels safely in meditation. Angels need to work with people as much as people need to work with angels, and the resulting partnership is surely destined.

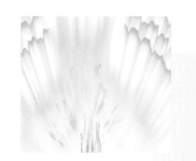

Archangel Uriel Meditation

THE RAINBOW BRIDGE TO
THE WORLD OF LIGHT

Uriel can be visualized with a rainbow brightness that is filled with gold. This meditation helps to build the rainbow bridge to the world of the angels, where you receive inspiration and help. It uses the colours of the spectrum and the colour of gold to deepen awareness of spiritual things. All the imagery you see shines through a golden radiance.

Prepare a meditation space with things that are the colour gold: Uriel's colour and the colour of fire and flame. Use a sheet of gold wrapping paper or a yellow cloth on a small table as your centrepiece. Find a gold- or yellow-coloured candle to light and use frankincense as incense or essential oil. Citrine crystals or tumblestones, or amber, will deepen the connection to Uriel.

Centre yourself with your breathing. Breathe slowly and gently, feeling the cool air against the tip of your nose as you breathe in, and the warm breath as you breathe out. Follow your breath down into the lungs, feel the expansion of your chest as you continue to breathe deeply but without strain. Visualize a blazing sun above your head, bathing you with rays of light. As you scan the golden light that surrounds and fills you, you realize that within the light can be seen all the colours of the rainbow. These colours are very subtle, pale and translucent.

At your feet and up your legs as far as your hips and pelvic area is the most beautiful shade of rose red. The sweet scent of rose fills your nostrils and surrounds you, giving you stability, strength and courage. Spend some time visualizing this beautiful shade of rose and inhaling the perfume.

Moving up your body, around your lower abdomen and navel, red rose changes to brilliant orange and fills your lower abdominal area and lower back with clear and beautiful orange light. The air is filled with the scent of oranges and mandarins and you absorb new energy, joy and creativity.

When you are ready, move your attention up towards the solar plexus and observe the brilliant orange gently shade into radiant yellow light. It surrounds the middle of your body around your waist and continues up to the sternum and ribcage. It shines and glows like the sun, bringing warmth, sunshine and courage into your life, dissolving all tiredness, weariness and depression.

Bring your attention upwards to your chest. Yellow gradually shades into green. At the centre of your chest, in the heart centre (chakra) is a beautiful rose of pale pink, surrounded by glossy green leaves. The heart chakra resonates to both green and pink. While a pink rose can represent spiritual love, green gives strength, adaptability and harmony. When you are feeling stressed, sitting in a beautiful park or garden surrounded by the greenery of the natural world assists relaxation. All these qualities are good for the sensitive chakra of the heart.

Breathe in the soft fragrance of the rose, feeling refreshed and harmonized by the green light with softest rose at its centre. You realize that the emotions of your heart have become tranquil and serene. You judge no one.

Now become aware of softest sapphire blue light,

surrounding your throat, like a scarf. It eases away any anger and aggression and you feel able to speak kindly and express yourself with truth, clarity and kindness. Sapphire blue gradually merges with indigo light, that wraps itself all around your forehead, the brow centre. It is like the colour of the night sky at dusk. You realize you are very intuitive and can trust the ideas and pictures that come into your mind and guide you to take the right action.

Above your head, you see violet with the sun's rays shining through it and are aware of the scent of violets, the bright, deep little flowers that grow wild or in gardens. You have opened to the highest spiritual guidance from your higher self, your soul. You have built the rainbow bridge from earth to heaven, the world of light.

Within the golden violet light, you see the form of Archangel Uriel. Mentally talk to him about any spiritual issues that concern you. This might be that you have lost your ideals or motivation for spending some regular time in meditation or living in an ethical way. Living in an ethical way means living your highest ideals. Whatever your difficulties, Uriel will help you to get back onto your spiritual path. He tells you that however unworthy you might feel because of things you perhaps have done in the past, you can always begin anew and he will support you. You feel surrounded and filled with golden rainbow light that encourages you to make new beginnings.

After thanking the archangel, you return to your everyday awareness by feeling the firmness of your body on the earth. Take three deep breaths and open your eyes.

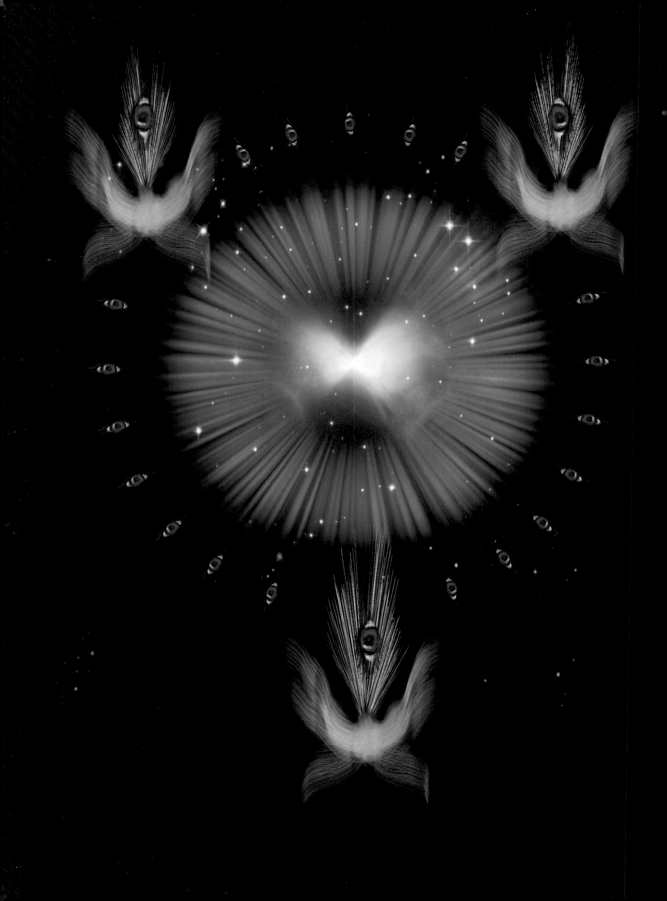

7.

Angels of Power, Wisdom and Love

Visualize an equilateral triangle, one point upward. All its sides are the same and its angles are exactly the same too. If you think of the apex, it represents your aspiration to angels and the Source of All-That-Is, the Creator. This triangle is like a ray of light and has a bright star of inspiration at its apex, sending inspiration into human life, radiating light into the darkness of materialism.

One side of the triangle says 'Power', one says 'Wisdom' and one says 'Love'.

THERE ARE three angels that work together with the symbol of the equilateral triangle. They are angels of balance and represent three qualities of power, wisdom and love that we can use to inspire us. Like the equilateral triangle, these qualities need to be kept in balance.

Power

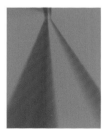

Power by itself, without wisdom, can corrupt and make people selfish and blind to the needs of others. There are many instances in the world where rulers and dictators take over a country and rule with cruelty and tyranny. This shows the extreme side of power, where (as the historian said) absolute power corrupts absolutely. In the business world, we find that laws are necessary to protect employees from workplace bullying and abuse. Even so, it is easy to feel depressed or inadequate when in the company of people who seem very confident and successful. Sometimes it feels difficult to speak out in meetings when others are full of ideas and it's hard to get a word in.

It's really good to generate positive thoughts about yourself, for the messages we send ourselves through our thoughts influence our bodies. The angels will help you do this, if you tune in to them, for the mere thought of telling yourself, 'I'm no good. I can never do anything right', or similar such things, will influence the cells of the body adversely. Suppressed anger can also cause health problems. This chapter will help you become confident and positive about yourself, for the right use of power includes being able to speak up truthfully and present your thoughts and ideas in such a way that you are respected. This means avoiding being passive and being aggressive equally. Positive thinking is spiritual alchemy, causing positive changes in the body and its cells.

Every thought and idea we have causes a reaction in the body. Two areas of the body, in particular, are involved in power and its use or abuse. One is the solar plexus. The endocrine gland associated with it is the pancreas. The chakra itself is known as the *manipura* chakra, a Sanskrit word meaning lustrous gem. It is involved in survival and our place in the world through work and relationships. In an imbalanced state it can cause someone to become a bully in the workplace or family, to overuse authority. It is equally imbalanced if someone is too shy and timid. When balanced, it helps with confidence and self-esteem and responsibility in decision-making. It's important not to give away our power by being too anxious to please, too passive or developing the 'poor me' syndrome and turning into a victim.

The solar plexus centre is also strengthened through deep breathing, as the movement of the ribs and the diaphragm in yoga breathing techniques develops strength in the muscles involved in breathing. There are many yoga breathing techniques, but one in particular is known as 'the victorious breath'.

HAND IN HAND WITH ANGELS

The Victorious Breath

Start by lying in the relaxation pose on the floor (see p. 51). Tune into your smooth, gentle, breathing first. Notice the rise and fall of the abdomen as you breathe. When you feel comfortably relaxed, slightly tighten the throat, so that when you breathe you make a slight hissing sound, as if it were a baby snoring. The hissing sound shouldn't be noisy. Breathe in and out through the nose and keep the mouth closed. Feel the ribs moving out to the side and at the back when you breathe in. Do this for as long as you feel comfortable, and then return to the relaxed gentle breath.

Sit up when you are ready. This breath helps to reduce stress and bring about a feeling of confidence when practised regularly. You can visualize your guardian angel helping you to develop strength and confidence when you breathe in this way.

A good affirmation to use is similar to the Yellow Ray one on p. 89:

I always know what to do and I always make the right decisions.

The other area of the body associated with power is the throat. The endocrine gland here is the thyroid and the chakra is the *visuddha* chakra. *Visuddha* (pronounced 'vishudda') means 'pure'. This chakra is associated with speaking truth in a pure, calm and clear way. When out of balance, the voice can be weak and throaty and sore throats can develop. Anger and rage occur at the other end of the range, when bad temper and impatience cause shouting—and sore throats and colds. This chakra can use personal power to create, and when it is used correctly, the voice resonates and is musical in speech, instead of either harsh and angry or weak and over-quiet.

An affirmation for the throat chakra and building

confidence is to repeat the word 'power' constantly to oneself, while visualizing the colour sapphire blue and focusing your attention in the throat and at the back of the tongue.

The Angel of Power has a message for those who can feel intimidated by the success of others when things don't seem to be working out and it's hard to express thoughts and feelings.

> **Remain empowered by your own ideas and suggestions. Your ideas are important and are part of a grand jewel of truth. Be confident in your own abilities. The jewel represents the combined ideas of all involved in a business or meeting. Each idea is like the facet of a jewel, which is polished by use. When neglected, it becomes dusty and loses its shine. Speak calmly and confidently and polish that jewel that is you.**

Love

The word 'love' is much overused and misunderstood. It brings joy and happiness and in its most altruistic definition refers to the unifying energy from the Source of All-That-Is. Love by itself, without wisdom, can become sentimental and smothering. The part of the body associated with pure

> *A Message from the Angel of Divine Love*
> **Remember to love yourself. You cannot love others if you cannot love yourself. Don't give in to guilt trips and feelings of guilt when you think you have done something wrong. Don't revisit scenes in your mind when people or things have upset you. Don't berate yourself for the things you consider mistakes. There are no mistakes. There are no failures. You learned something from the experience. When you come to a pothole in the road, go around it. Find another way. And remember the forgiving power of Divine Love and forgive yourself. Then you can be free to be healthy and happy. Love is the healer for all ills. Doing what you love is your healer.**

A while ago, we were waiting for a flight home from holiday in the Canary Islands. We felt rested and refreshed from our time in the warm sunshine, sandy beaches and blue sea. The plane was delayed and everyone in the queue was grumbling about it. Not one person talked about the wonderful holiday they had, the beautiful weather or the beauty of the island. The grumbles collected around the people like a dark, damp cloud of depression. It's hard to remain cheerful when surrounded by gloom. We can then use our power of love to say silently affirmations like 'peace', 'love', or 'calm'. This is not a state of denial, but the use of the creative power of affirmation and visualization to create a better atmosphere around us. On another occasion, a family got into our compartment in a train and were arguing and grumbling. Quietly sitting there, I repeated silently the words 'divine love' over and over again while visualizing them in light. Before long the family were chatting cheerfully.

love is the heart chakra, *anahata chakra*. The word *anahata* means 'unstruck', in the sense of being pure and unhurt. When we can overcome the grief and hurt in which human life itself involves us, we may reach a state of openness and trust. Grumbling and gossip can close down the chakra and it becomes a place of unfair judgment.

The thymus gland is sometimes known as the higher heart chakra. The heart chakra is in the centre of the chest and the higher heart chakra, the thymus gland, is higher up, towards the collarbone. The thymus gland produces T-cells and helps the functioning of the immune system.

Here is an affirmation for you:

I do what I love and I love what I do.

Overleaf, there is a meditation with the Angel of Divine Love.

A Meditation with the Angel of Divine Love

Begin your meditation in the usual way. When you feel still and centred, visualize yourself standing before a magnificent door opening into a library. Design it mentally as the most beautiful door you can create. At the door, there is an angel wearing robes of clear rose pink. She asks you for the password to open the door. The password is to radiate a ray of light and love from your heart chakra.

The door opens and you go into a room. It is very dusty and neglected. You realize that it represents your heart chakra and any upsets you have tried to forget. Create any cleaning materials that you need to dust and polish the room. Dust the furniture, polish the floor and clean the windows. There are also French windows leading to a delightful garden. Open them and allow pure fresh air to enter the room. Look around the room. The furniture is attractive and there is a comfortable sofa for you.

Wisdom

Wisdom is not the same thing as knowledge. Knowledge is learned from books or teachers or other modern sources like the Internet. Wisdom comes from our spirit or higher self.

Many angels work to bring us wisdom. You might think of them as information angels, but their information is not the same as the information found in a book. Wisdom angels are the librarians of the angelic kingdom and will communicate through meditation. They might give direct information and

The Angel of Divine Love encourages you to explore the room. Decide how you want it to be and create the furniture and furnishings you like the best, in your favourite colours. The angel then shows you a little silver box on a shelf in the corner. It is tarnished and needs polishing. Clean and polish the box. You realize there is a golden key on a golden chain around your neck. It opens the box. Inside you see your heart, which has been locked away for protection.

What does it look like? The angel asks you if you want to keep it locked and hidden or keep it open. You can decide what you want to do. If you decide to take the heart out of the box and put it in your chest, the angel will help you. Sit in the room and look out into the garden, which is a safe place to go in meditation when you need to. The Angel of Divine Love will always be there for you.

When power and love combine with wisdom, it develops the spiritual alchemy whereby hard materialism can be transmuted into gold, the golden light of spirituality.

be regarded like a muse and fill you with wisdom information that you need for a particular project. They might also guide you to books, films or songs, or even dreams, which provide what you need to know. Their function is to give you the information you ask for. Invite them into your life, for they will love to help you. Archangel Raziel is known as the Angel of Wisdom (see the Yellow Ray section, pp. 89–91). You can use the meditation of the library above to get in touch with any of the angels of wisdom, as well as Archangel Raziel himself.

A Meditation to Balance Power, Wisdom and Love

Visualize yourself sitting in a pyramid or tent of light. It is like an equilateral triangle with the apex exactly above your head. On your right side stands the Angel of Power. It has masculine energy. This is the energy you should use in everyday life when you need to get things done. Its colour is vibrant clear red. It tells you to call on its help when you need strength and power to help you in your life and work. Visualize yourself being filled with the colour red, bringing strength and courage.

On your left side stands the Angel of Love. Its energy is feminine and its colour is pale rose pink. She reminds you that you can use her energy to keep your power in balance. You don't need to give your power away by being submissive, but you don't need to be aggressive either. You can use pink to tone down the shade of red.

Behind you stands the Angel of Wisdom. Its colour is yellow and it tells you that power and love in balance become wisdom. You can blend the three colours together to make gold, the colour of spiritual wisdom. A peace rose with its gold petals tipped with rose is also an ideal symbol of the love and wisdom that produces power.

Use this visualization when you need to find a balance between difficult choices. It helps you to work with the power of love rather than the love of power.

Draw a triangle and label each of the sides with one attribute—wisdom, love or power. Write along each side of the triangle any words that may help you to become wise, loving and powerful. Power is best thought of as being true to yourself, and not being forceful or bossy.

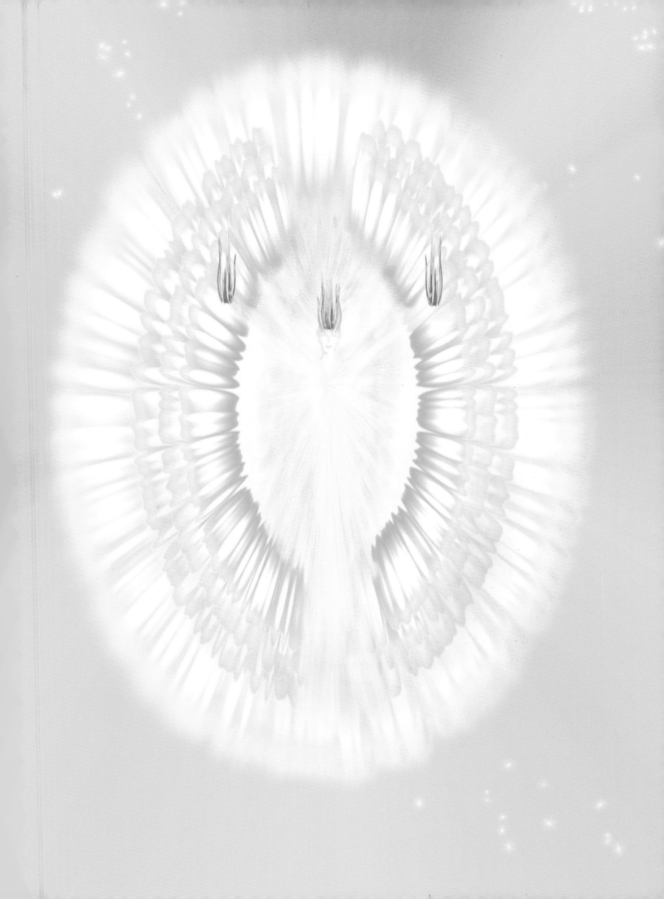

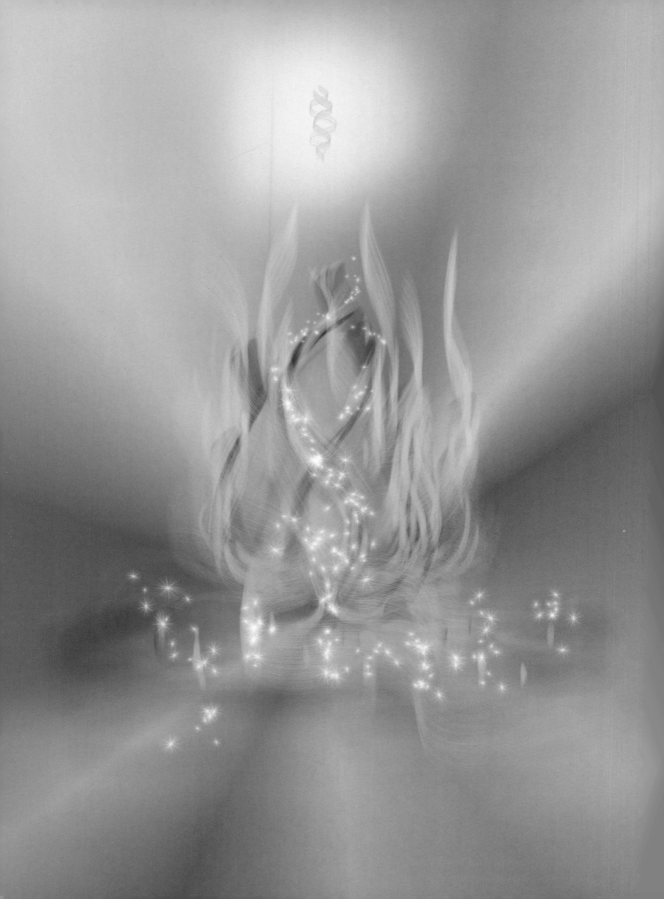

8.
Angels of
Inspiration

THIS CHAPTER begins with a number of different stories and meditations. Sometimes we seem to go through periods of frustration and we lose our inspiration. We may feel that we can't see the future and feel frustrated because we don't know what to do. Angels are always there to inspire us and encourage us.

I have been fortunate to see and work with angels for many years. I come from a family tradition where angels were seen and talked about. My first really powerful experience with angels came on retreat in 1976. Having been involved in the White Eagle Lodge healing work for a couple of years, I was sitting in a healing service in the White Temple in Hampshire, England, waiting for it to begin. Suddenly, everything faded from view and the only things I could see were two immense angels, as tall as the building itself. I saw them in profile, kneeling on each side of the altar flame, with hands in prayer.

The light on the altar was also magnified many times and the angels were enormous. The walls and ceiling of the building had totally disappeared in light. The angels didn't say anything, and the vision faded as quickly as it had appeared. I felt very emotional and remained so for several days. For no apparent reason that I knew, I would keep bursting into tears. Perhaps it was the effect of the vision, perhaps the effect of going on retreat, but this experience really seemed to change my life.

When I was at home again, some colleagues asked me to teach them yoga. I began to teach yoga classes and then to train yoga teachers and it was then that my business, 'KEYS', was founded, actually in 1984. We called it KEYS because doing the courses opens new doors in your life. In 1993, I was able to leave the teaching profession to work full time with Roy in our own business.

Passing into the Light

Angels are always with us when we have finished our time on earth and it is time to pass on. Ever since my mother's vision, which follows, we have referred to death as going home.

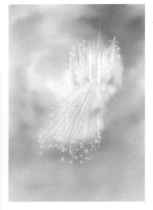

In 1963 my father, Stan, died suddenly, about midnight. I was newly married and lived in another town and we didn't have a phone then, so my mother, Nancy, couldn't contact me until I was at work the next day. My parents had been very happily married for nearly twenty-five years. Nobody could ever imagine them apart. Truly, they had never been known to argue. After the doctor had been and formalities completed, Nancy went to spend the rest of the night with friends. She lay sleepless. Suddenly the walls of the room seemed to dissolve into light. Shafts of light and colour flooded into the room. Shining figures of angels were seen moving up and down as if on a ladder. She was aware of preparations for a celebration and there was a feeling of intense happiness. She felt the happiness and joy of the spirit world and she could hear voices talking excitedly, telling each other that Stan was coming home and they must get a party ready to welcome him home. This vision comforted her in the early days of bereavement and gave us all an unshakeable belief in the continuity of life beyond death. Angels are always present at death, ready to carry the soul into the new life.

An interesting coincidence accompanies this story and demonstrates the law of synchronicity. When I began to teach angel workshops in 1998, it was this story about angels I liked to tell when we were sharing our stories. I used the version from the book where my mother's story had been published, It was *Miracles,* by Bettine Pickles, who was a friend of hers.

After the first workshop, I was going through some papers

HAND IN HAND WITH ANGELS

of my mother's and I found the original handwritten account of the story, which she had written for Bettine to put in the book. My mother had been in the world of light for about ten years at the time and I had no idea that I even had this account, but I am sure that it was the angels who led me to find it. I have my own story to tell, though, about my mother's passing.

My mother passed away quite suddenly in 1988, having suffered a stroke, followed by two weeks in a coma in the local hospital. Before the final phone call came from the hospital, about 10.30 pm, I was very aware of the change in the atmosphere at home. It became almost electric and was particularly noticeable in my meditation room. The light was very bright. I knew angels were there. Then the phone rang. The hospital asked us to return there as my mother had taken a turn for the worse. She passed away around midnight.

While she was in the hospital I would awaken early each morning and see her with my inner vision. She was with my father. He was rowing them in a boat across a beautiful lake. Each day, they would be further away. After two weeks, one morning when I woke up, I heard a woman's voice singing to me. She was singing one of the solos from Handel's *Messiah*, 'Rejoice, rejoice greatly, O daughter of Zion'. My mother was a singer and had sung the soprano solos from *The Messiah* many times, and I knew she was telling me not to worry but to be glad for her that she and my father were reunited after twenty-five years.

If your family are facing sickness or death, be confident in the presence and help of angels that support you. Think of them and they will be able to come closer to you. They will sustain you during the weeks and months following bereavement, when you maybe long for the friendship and companionship of your family and friends who have gone on before.

The Angel of Peace

I had the meditation on the following page at one of our group meetings. If you are interested in numerology and the secret power of numbers, the date was also very interesting. The number 11 is a master number and also represents a gateway, as it is like two pillars. The date of this meditation was 1.11.01. Of course, Remembrance Day itself is 11.11 (plus the year). In numerology, you don't reduce these numbers, which remain 11. I use visualizations like this whenever I hear depressing news on radio and television, to counteract the fear and negativity that such news can spread.

The Angel of Happiness

The Angel of Happiness has a message for you.

> Remember how happy you feel when the sun shines after a dull, stormy or cloudy day. Remember a place where you love to be. Remember being in the warm sunshine there. Is it in your garden? Is it in a beautiful park or the garden of a stately home? Is it in the mountains, the forest, or by the sea on a soft, sandy beach?
>
> Remember the sounds you can hear in your favourite place. Can you hear the birds singing and the insects buzzing, or the sound of the seashore? Can you hear the gentle splashing of waves on a beach? Can you hear the sound of a gentle breeze as it blows in the branches and bushes?
>
> Remember what you can see. Is the sky a brilliant shade of blue? Are there butterflies that have iridescent shades and colours on their wings? What can you smell? Think of all the sweet natural scents of your special place, like the salty tang of the sea, scents of flowers, the sweet, fresh air.
>
> Create all the things that make you happy with your inner vision and keep them in your mind. Remember that in our world 'enjoyment' means 'joy is meant'. Always be joyful and spread joy wherever you go. Every day, do something that brings you joy and brings joy to others.

Write down ten memories that make you happy. Then choose one of them and draw yourself as a stick person and write words around yourself noting what happened that made it so joyous. You might remember the weather, people, places, or scenery.

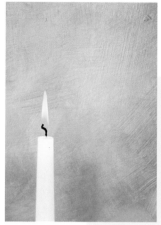

A Meditation on the Angel of Peace

Sit quietly in front of a candle and use flowers and incense, or your favourite crystal. Any or all of these enhance the spiritual atmosphere. Begin your meditation by doing a few minutes of gentle breathing. Feel every breath as it comes and goes.

When you feel centred and relaxed, begin to visualize a beautiful shining jewel in your heart chakra. It sparkles and flashes like a diamond and changes colour as the light is reflected. It fills the whole of your heart and lungs, and then your whole being (both physical and spiritual) is renewed in its spiritual light. As this drop of diamond-like dew expands, it begins to send out rays of light.

Continuing the meditation, see a brilliant angel within the light. It is silver, blue and pink. Its aura covers the whole earth. See the planet contained within the heart centre of this great being. As you continue to radiate light from your heart centre, the Angel of Peace gathers up the rays of light and scatters them like raindrops. They fall into the hearts of those who are engaged in conflict and war and they start to make changes for the better as they begin to feel more peaceful and caring.

Now the angel holds aloft a beautiful shining crystal bowl. It gathers into the bowl the light you are sending it, together with the light of all those who meditate for peace. As this light fills the bowl it overflows like water, running like a waterfall down onto the earth, and streams along the ground, forming a river of light and peace. As it flows along the ground, it transforms and purifies all darkness and negativity, before joining streams and rivers and then an ocean of peace.

Just as the oceans and seas are filled with water drop by drop, so we change the world thought by thought. The Angel of Peace gathers up all prayers for peace sent by light workers right across the earth and radiates them to the places where they are needed.

I hope you tried the Attunement Activity on p. 130, which suggested drawing a stick person surrounded by joy. Using the memory that you drew, try the visualization that follows, which begins with the memory of joyful times. It is a traditional meditation from the east. It is reputed to bring about healing as well as happiness. It is called 'the Inner Smile'.

Visualize each part of the body and smile into it. Invite the Angels of Joy and Happiness to be with you. This is said to be a powerful healing practice when done regularly. It can be used with any qualities you want to develop and the angels associated with them, such as the angels of joy, healing, peace, patience, or freedom. This meditation makes use of positive thinking and circulation of prana, or chi, the life-force, to each part of the body. Happy (inner) smiling!

The Inner Smile

Begin your meditation in the usual way, sitting comfortably on a chair or on the floor. Begin to observe your breathing for a few minutes until your mind becomes quiet and still. Then begin to recall the event that you drew about that makes you smile and feel happy. Bring into your conscious mind the feelings that you remember and allow yourself to smile. Invite the Angels of Joy and Happiness to be with you and visualize them in joyful colours sitting beside you.

Relax your forehead, which houses the brow centre (chakra), and let your inner or third eye open. Allow your smiling energy to fill your inner eye and then your physical eyes. Then let this energy flow up your forehead and over your head, down the sides of your head into your ears and all the facial muscles. Feel your face relaxing.

Follow the smiling energy down your face, neck and throat and into your shoulders and chest. Feel it flowing into the thymus gland, which sits just behind the sternum above the heart. Visualize it opening and vibrating like a beautiful flower, as it becomes filled with loving, smiling

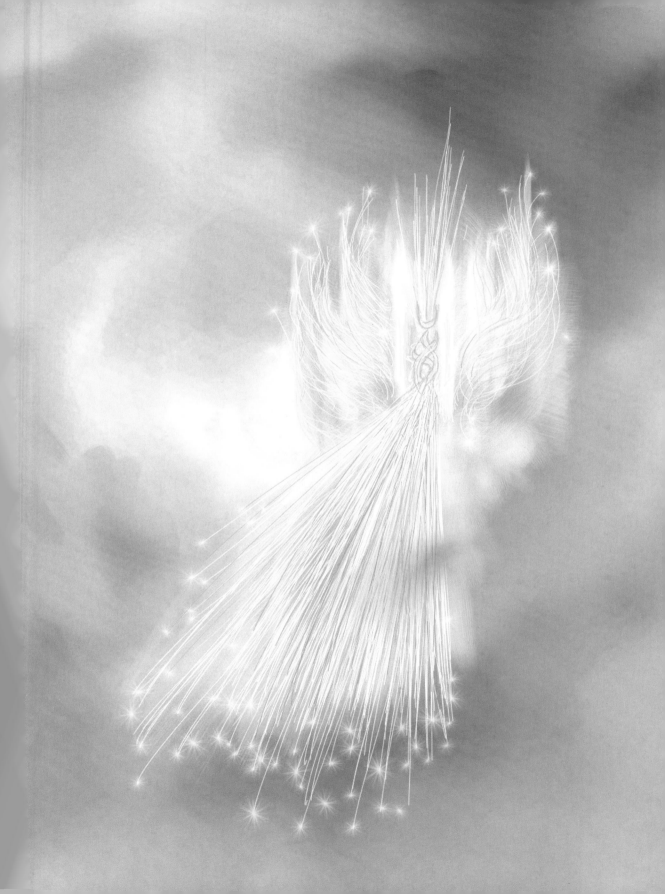

9.

Angels and Crystals

> Crystals are born deep inside the earth and remain hidden there for aeons. They are creations of loveliness. They represent the beauty and healing properties of Mother Earth, Gaia, and are her gift to you. A clear quartz crystal will help you to have crystal clear intentions. Their colours and vibrations enhance your work with angels. The colours resonate with the seven rays and heal and complement the connection with angels.
>
> (Words from the Crystal Deva)

CRYSTALS—by which we mean beautiful rock crystals, including many gems—are millions of years old. They were 'born' deep within the earth and there are many varieties and colours. Each crystal has a definite atomic structure and many geometric shapes are found, such as the prism with six triangular faces forming a point as with the quartz crystal. Since ancient times, gems and crystals have been used as spiritual symbols and talismans and worn or carried for their healing properties. Crystals are admired for their beauty and can be used to enhance the environment as office paperweights, or around the home or workplace as ornaments which improve the vibrations and beauty of the area. Crystals are reputed to disperse electromagnetic smog from cell phones, television sets and computers.*

Once someone makes contact with and uses the universal

*The Crystal Bible, by Judy Hall

energy of crystals, they are using the energy from which the universe itself is constructed. For this reason, crystal energy should always be used for the highest good of all beings and never for selfish purposes. Having the right intention for the use of minerals and crystals means that they will begin to work with the higher consciousness of the individual, and the angels, thus beginning transformation and healing of the person, their environment and the planet.

The energy in crystals derives from what is known as the piezoelectric effect ('the linear electromechanical interaction between the mechanical and the electrical state in crystalline materials', *Wikipedia*), and it links with the complex electromagnetic system in the human body. Crystals are said to be perfect electromagnetic conductors of energy. Crystal healing is part of a wider range of vibrational healing methods such as acupuncture, homeopathy, flower remedies and colour healing. It may restore balance and promote a sense of well-being, reducing the effects of stress.

When quartz crystals are subject to pressure, they produce a measurable electrical voltage. The ancients knew this. Archaeologists have found deposits of quartz crystals and pyrite crystals together in ancient campsites. They were used to light fires. When the pyrite is struck against the point of the quartz, it produces a flame and can light a fire. I had definite evidence of this recently when one of my quartz crystals fell on the floor and broke. I took it into the garden where I put broken crystals. On the way, it dropped again onto the stone path. A great flash of light shone from it. I was quite surprised at how bright it was. Computers and digital watches and other electronic devices utilize a slice or piece of quartz.

There is an angel responsible for the mineral kingdom, as well as other angels that have a particular connection with each gemstone. The highest purpose of crystal angels is in their service to humanity, removing pain and suffering. A *deva* is another word for an angelic being and it means 'shining one' (see p. 17); devas are particularly linked with manifestations such as crystals. Thus the universal crystal deva works with crystal healers and therapists who use them to bring healing energies into their practice space.

This deva urges people to work in an ethical way with crystals. We all know that gemstone mining can be influenced by greed and dishonesty. Used responsibly, crystals and gemstones bring higher vibrations into our lives and assist in transmuting past conditions and transforming our lives and our health and wellbeing. Crystals and gemstones resonate with the highest qualities of the healers and therapists who use them. If crystals are used to enhance the energy of a workplace or office, it is good to remember to cleanse them from the negative vibrations they can pick up from the environment they are in. Some gemstones, like black tourmaline, smoky quartz and blue kyanite, don't need cleansing, as they are self-cleansing. Black tourmaline is particularly good for dispersing negative energy. I keep pieces by the television and the computer to keep the energy in the house clean and pure.

There are several ways to cleanse and purify old, stale, energy from crystals. Some can be rinsed or soaked in pure filtered or mineral water. They can be placed on sunny windowsills or in the light of the full moon. A quick method of cleansing that a therapist or healer can use between clients is to sound a singing bowl or tingshas, the little cymbals made from seven sacred metals. Before using crystals, dedicate them to the highest good. A suitable dedication is this:

> Highest Creative Source (*or any spiritual name of God you like to use*), I thank you for this semi-precious stone. Please activate all its good vibrations for my highest good and may these good vibrations render useless all harmful influences around us all. And so it is.

A crystal will tell you the information it has stored within it and how to use it. Although there are many crystal reference books and encyclopaedias now available with information on crystal use, you can enhance that information by meditating with the crystal or gemstone and the individual deva of the particular one.

People often ask how they can choose the right crystal for their purpose. It is the crystal that chooses you! This has

and polished like glass.

Now you see a beautiful, shining being standing in front of you. She is the crystal deva. She is here to ask you if you would like to work more closely with angels and crystals. She asks you if you will work with them in a responsible way. You promise not to be acquisitive and greedy, but to work with crystals for the highest good of all humanity, to bring about healing and transformation both to people and the planet. Then the deva asks you to choose a colour you need right now. Face the wall of the crystal temple that is your chosen colour. Bathe in the coloured light that showers all over you and around you. Breathe it in and feel it fill every part of you, bringing the healing qualities that you need from the colour.

When you have finished this colour breathing, stand in the centre of the crystal where all colours blend into pure light. Stand in a ray of pure light that shines all around you. Fill yourself with light as you breathe in. When you breathe out, radiate it to people and places that need peace and healing. You can use this affirmation to help you.

As you breathe in, silently say, 'I breathe in light'.
Before breathing out, say, 'I am light'.
As you breathe out, say, 'I breathe out light'.

Finish by thanking the crystal deva. Leave the crystal cave through the door that you entered. It is now time to leave this special place, but you can return any time you wish.

You can also use this meditation to find out about a particular crystal you want to work with. Substitute the crystal you are investigating for the large quartz.

Special Crystals that Enhance your Clear Connection with Angels

The chapter about the Seven Rays (p. 77) contains a lot of useful information about using colour, crystals and angels for your life, work or healing. There are also other crystals that particularly make it easier to meditate more deeply and connect to angels. Angelite and celestite are particular crystals that deepen the connection to angels. There are old fairy stories that talk about beautiful princesses or heroines who are sent on special quests. The ones who are kind and helpful find that when they speak, pearls, diamonds and roses fall from their lips. Metaphorically speaking, this is the kind of effect that comes from working with angelic gemstones. Speech becomes gentler and you are able to speak truthfully in a kind way, which is more helpful and non-critical to the listener. Kyanite is a crystal that is linked particularly with Archangel Michael.

ANGELITE: Communication with angels

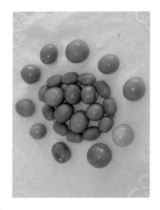

Angelite is a beautiful blue gemstone with a white exterior. Stories are that it was first found after the Harmonic Convergence of 1987 (see p. 168). That was a special event when the human race collectively decided to go for spiritual growth and development. It changed everything on the planet. This is shown by the phenomenal growth of interest in personal and spiritual development, healing, reiki, crystals and meditation that has happened since that time. An Internet search will find you information about it. On the internet, the Wikipedia article on angelite is particularly helpful.

Angelite resonates with the throat chakra and third-eye centre, thus enabling the user to connect with angels and higher beings. It soothes the throat chakra after overuse or misuse—such as anger, rage or resentment. It helps to bring beauty and clarity to the words you use. Here is an affirmation:

I am open to messages from my guardian angels and all angels of light.

Use in Healing:
Like all angel gemstones, it brings an angelic note to speech.

CELESTITE: Communication with higher worlds, beings of light, spiritual dimensions, access to divine healing.

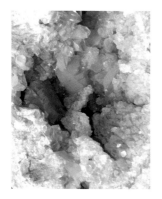

Celestite is another pale blue gemstone, but much more translucent than angelite. It is often more grey and can be almost white. It likes to be in a shady corner as the colour might fade in strong light. It is very successful in enhancing the connection to angels of light, your guardian angel and accessing higher spiritual information. Clusters of celestite are good in the bedroom, therapy room or meditation room to cleanse the environment, as its energy radiates out in many directions.

Affirmation:

I now access my ability to communicate with spirit and angels.

Meditation with angels and higher beings is enhanced by using angelite and celestite alone or with other gemstones. These stones can enhance any of the meditations found in this book.

KYANITE: Crossing inner bridges to the world of Archangel Michael and the archangelic realm, leading to inner spiritual growth.

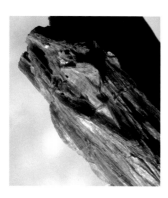

Kyanite is usually blue, although it can be found in other colours such as pink, green, yellow, grey or black. It is formed of striated blades that have a pearly sheen. The blue variety seems to be the most easily found and usually comes from Brazil. The one in the picture looks as though it has an angel in it!

Use in Healing:
Blue kyanite can heal energy blocks in the aura and emotional blocks between people. It can clear the energy field. It assists

in lucid dreams when put under the pillow at night. It is good on the heart chakra, throat and third eye or to hold for meditation. It helps people to speak truthfully in a clear and balanced way.

Archangel Michael uses a flashing sword to cut unhealthy ties that no longer serve you. Kyanite blades are like the flashing sword. Hold kyanite in meditation to help cut unhealthy cords with people, relationships, places and stuck situations. You can use kyanite with the Archangel Michael meditation on pp. 82–4. Lie in relaxation and place a piece of kyanite gemstone over the heart chakra or the third eye or hold it in your dominant hand. Tune in to your breathing. Notice each breath as it comes and goes. Then direct each breath into the gemstone. As you attune more and more to the kyanite you may see the form of Archangel Michael more clearly before you in the meditation.

Affirmation:

I now cross inner bridges and open to the angelic realms. I reach Archangel Michael for guidance and truth. This is released to me in perfect and harmonious ways, under grace and in divine right order.

Devic Temple Crystals

Devic Temple crystals are part of the family of master quartz crystals. They can be recognized by reading the inclusions seen in the world inside the crystal and reading the other markings on its body and faces. They are often cloudy or milky in appearance. These crystals can be used as temple sites by otherworldly angelic beings or devas. Only devas devoted to pure white light may enter the crystals and cross the threshold between the two worlds. They enhance communication between the two worlds and a magical presence prevails. The harmonic vibration of these quartz temples lifts the veils between the two worlds and spiritual energies infiltrate the environment.

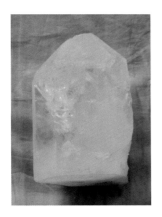

A Devic Temple crystal can become a living altar through which a guide, an angel or a master from beyond the veil can see into the heart, mind and soul of the crystal keeper who will meditate with and use it. According to the talents and special gifts of the crystal keeper, the deva dwelling within the crystal can be used to enhance them. This can be done through meditation and by carrying the crystal for the particular purpose it is for. It needs to be specially dedicated for its use and when at rest can be kept on an altar or in a special container, such as a silk purse or a piece of silk. A Devic Temple can become a personal shrine where the deva can assist those who use it.

Create an altar for the crystal by using incense or smudge, fresh flowers and a white candle. Make some kind of personal offering each time you call on the deva. It needs to be something close to your heart and the purpose for which you wish to use the crystal. It should be the same each time. You could sing, chant, intone or play a musical instrument. Then close your eyes and go within. Call the deva that you feel drawn to. Then open your eyes and gaze into the crystal. Keep your mind clear and your heart open. The guidance may be indirect.

The altar needs to be kept activated daily to continue to work with the devas. They are master teachers working through master crystals to teach self-mastery. They do not want to build a psychic relationship. They will direct you straight to the heart of God.

One of my friends bought one to enhance her work with music and playing her violin. Over time, she had greater insights into ways she could improve her understanding of the violin, how she could improve her music when playing it and what the crystal could do.

DANBURITE: The Karmic Cleanser—change, leaving behind the past

Danburite is a clear striated crystal with a diamond-shaped cross section and a termination shaped like a wedge. Metaphysically, it is an important stone and the clearest examples are found in Mexico. Danburite has a very high spiritual vibration and stimulates the third eye and clears and opens the crown chakra and balances it with the heart chakra. It opens chakras in the etheric body that are above the crown, enabling a clearer connection with the angelic realms. Its brilliance is not from Planet Earth but from cosmic light. It smoothes the path ahead. Wearing it brings serenity and eternal wisdom. Look out for danburite with a Buddha formation within the crystal, a form which draws enlightenment to you.

Danburite is the crystal to bring about profound changes and to leave behind the past. Its ability in cleansing means that it can clear karmic miasms and mental patterns from past lives. Keep a danburite crystal by the bed or under the pillow or somewhere else in the bedroom to aid lucid dreaming and stimulate spiritual dreams and to bring inner guidance. Danburite brings the purity of the trinity of wisdom, love and power and a connection with the angelic kingdom.

Use in Healing:
Use for the liver, gallbladder, allergies and detoxifying at all levels. Make it into a gem essence or aura spray and note down your meditations in a journal.

Angel:
The angel of danburite is a beautiful translucent one, with a rainbow aura of light radiating all around him. The lord of karma has the name Metatron.

Affirmation:

I thank the angels of karma for the release and cleansing of all negative karma under grace and in divine right order so that angelic healing will manifest in my life.

Meditation with Danburite

Lie in relaxation and place a danburite crystal on the heart chakra or third eye. Tune in to your breathing. Notice each breath as it comes and goes. Then direct each breath into the crystal. Visualize the crystal growing bigger until you are able to feel yourself inside it. You find yourself inside a magnificent temple of light. The light is very pure and clear. There is a radiance as if from the sun, and all the colours of the spectrum are seen scintillating and sparkling in the aura of the temple.

You see a beautiful angel, the Angel of Danburite. He enfolds you in his aura of light, the light you see inside the crystal temple. You become aware of a circle of angels surrounding you, pointing danburite crystals towards you. Breathe in this pure light and feel it permeating all through you, dissolving away any issues you know about and also any you are not aware of.

Continue with this vision until you feel ready to return to your everyday awareness, being careful to notice any inner guidance or inspiration. Know that the crystal is aiding the process of enlightenment, of heightened awareness of spiritual growth and wisdom. Then, when you are ready, breathe yourself back to your everyday consciousness. Feel yourself growing larger and see a grounding cord from your feet into the centre of the earth. Take your time.

LARIMAR: Peace, serenity and tranquillity

Larimar is only found in the Dominican Republic, and is said to resonate with dolphins, Atlantis and goddess energy. Many people consider Mother Mary to be an angel, and she is known as the Queen of Angels. Larimar is an excellent gemstone for those who need an angelic and motherly reconnection. It is a beautiful blue colour, like the sky or the sea. It was discovered during the latter part of the twentieth century. It gets its name from the daughter of the man who discovered it, Larissa, and *mar*, the Spanish for sea. Its colours shade from blue through pale green to white. Pictures and patterns, like angels and birds, often reveal themselves within the gemstone.

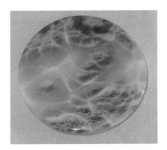

Affirmation:

> I am at peace. God is with me.

Meditation with Larimar

Lie in the relaxation pose (p. 51) on the floor. Place a piece of larimar on the heart centre. Tune in to your breathing. Breathe slowly and deeply. Be aware of the breath entering your chest and heart chakra. Visualize yourself lying on a warm sandy beach. You can see the blue sky above you and hear the gentle lapping of the waves on the beach not far away. You breathe in the peace and serenity of the blue sky and sea.

You see a beautiful blue angel in front of you. There are many shades of blue, ranging from deep sky blue to palest ice blue. The angel's aura surrounds you in blue light and you feel utterly peaceful and serene. Your breath seems to follow the rhythm of the lapping waves and your breath flows in and out to their rhythm. Stay in that scene as long as you like before concluding your relaxation.

Angel:
Mother Mary, the Holy Mother.

Use in Healing:
Larimar diffuses and cools anger and rage and it works well on the throat chakra. It is a good gemstone for singers and people who need to use their voice in their work, like actors and teachers, and also for healers and therapists. It is a good stone for women during and after pregnancy. It is beneficial to wear it often as a pendant, where it lies between the heart and throat chakras to soothe and balance them.

MOLDAVITE: The star-born stone of transformation, it speeds up spiritual development

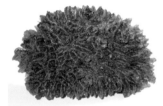

Moldavite is a dark green stone and is a form of tektite, created when a large meteorite crashed to earth in what is now the Bohemian Plateau of the Czech Republic. The heat of the impact caused the surrounding rocks to metamorphose and be scattered over a wide area. Scientists disagree about its origin. Some say it was formed by terrestrial rock that melted with the heat. Others say it may be a form of volcanic glass of lunar origin. A third theory is that it was vaporized gas, which solidified on impact. However, whichever theory is correct, because the energy of moldavite is both earthly and non-terrestrial, it is called 'the star-born stone of transformation'.

It connects the user with the angelic kingdom, as moldavite is considered to have been a meteorite that landed in the earth's atmosphere, bringing with it the energies of angels and otherworldly beings. It has its own vast cosmic angel.

Use moldavite carefully until you are familiar with it. It can leave you 'spaced out'!

Affirmation:

I now release all limiting thought-patterns. I am transformed in perfect and harmonious ways.

Use in Healing:

Moldavite is especially good for 'star children'. These are people who believe they are not of the earth, but are incarnated here for a special mission at this particular time. It has been claimed that moldavite was the gemstone from which the Holy Grail was formed. A legend states that the cup of the Last Supper had a moldavite gemstone on it. In ancient India it was known as *agni mani*, fire pearl. It was considered very valuable and rare. The energy of moldavite is enhanced by the use of other gems, especially quartz. It is a high-vibration stone, which enables the user to connect with angels, and unfolds visions of the past or the future. It can cause a warm wave to sweep over the body, which can be seen on the face as blushing. This is known as the moldavite flush. The green colour of moldavite indicates a resonance with the heart chakra.

Archangels: Ariel, Raphael, Raziel.

Meditation with Moldavite

Lie in relaxation and place a moldavite crystal on the heart chakra, where it forms a bridge to the gateway into the heart. Tune in to your breathing. Notice each breath as it comes and goes. Then direct each breath into the crystal. You begin to feel surrounded by a soft green light. It brings about a feeling of warmth and harmony. It softly dissolves away any old emotional wounds. You become aware of a vast angelic being, the Angel of Moldavite. You may ask the angel to connect you with any ascended master or archangel, or any guides and angels of your own. Ask to be shown a vision of what you need to do for your spiritual development or transformation.

Continue with this vision until you feel ready to return to your everyday awareness. Then when you are ready, breathe yourself back to your everyday consciousness.

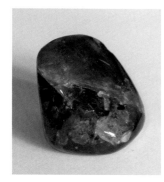

Iolite is a vision-prophecy stone. It is safe to carry or wear it but should only be placed on the third eye if the other chakras are all in balance, as it can cause overstimulation. It is a vision-quest guide and a guardian when you go on inner or outer journeys of self-exploration. It awakens inner wisdom and clears confusion about your life purpose. It is a stone of the Violet Ray. Iolite is a rare stone, often only available from specialist shops. It is also found as iolite-sunstone, in which form it inspires its user in artistic and creative pursuits.

Use iolite carefully until you are familiar with it. Don't put it over the third eye if in any doubt. Do some colour breathing before you meditate. Colour breathing balances the chakras. Sit in your favourite meditation pose and begin to attune to your breathing. Then visualize the seven colours of the spectrum in turn. Do three breaths visualizing red, then three breaths for each of the following colours: orange, yellow, green, blue, indigo and violet. Conclude with three breaths of white light. Then continue with the mediation given.

I acknowledge my own intuition and power to know, which now manifests in my life in perfect and harmonious ways, under grace and in divine right order.

Archangels: Raziel and Zadkiel, according to my guidance. I have not been able to confirm this from any other source. Zadkiel is the archangel of the Violet Ray.

Meditation with Iolite

Lie in relaxation and hold an iolite crystal, or, if you are sure, place over the third eye on the brow (*ajna*) chakra. Tune in to your breathing. Notice each breath as it comes and goes. Then direct each breath into the crystal. You may ask to be connected with the Master 'R' or Archangel Zadkiel, of the Violet Ray, or any guides and angels of your own. You may use the violet fire of cleansing and transmutation first if you wish. Then ask to know your true self, beyond the outer personality. Insights may come during this meditation, or may come in dreams, lucid dreams or at another time.

Continue with this vision until you feel ready to return to your everyday awareness. When you are ready, breathe yourself back to consciousness of the physical world. Create a grounding cord from your feet into the centre of the earth. Take some time to feel sure you are not too 'floaty'. Drink some water to ground yourself. Write down whatever you remember in your meditation journal.

PETALITE: Serenity, opening to higher worlds

Petalite is a very clear, colourless gemstone, although it can be found in pink or yellow forms. It is a very spiritual stone and a visionary one. It is a very good gemstone to help you to clarify your higher spiritual path. As well as being a high-vibrational stone, it also helps to keep you grounded, so that you can bring spiritual knowledge into practical, everyday life and work. Petalite is 'brilliant' to use for meditation. Wearing it or carrying it every day helps to keep you calm and centred and able to cope with stress. It is usually found in small pieces only. Sometimes it is possible to find small pieces of petalite jewellery, but they are usually expensive.

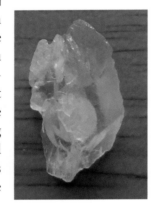

Angel:
the Angel of Light, or any angel the user wishes.

Affirmation:

> I now connect with the higher realms.
> I enable spiritual knowledge to permeate my life.
> I am filled with pure light that dissolves all shadows within me.

HAND IN HAND WITH ANGELS

Meditation with Petalite

Lie in the yoga relaxation pose, *savasana* (see p. 51). Place a piece of petalite on either the heart or third eye chakra, or place one on the floor behind the crown chakra so it is just touching it. Attune to your breathing and breathe the pure white light energy of the Angel of Light down your body. Take the light down to your feet, and gradually fill your whole body with light. If you have any emotional difficulties, like stress at work, spend some time working on bringing light into the situation.

Is there a place in your body where you feel the stress? If there is, send a special concentration there. Ask the Angel of Light to bring light into the situation. This is very beneficial to release issues like workplace bullying. Thank the Angel of Light. When you have finished, have a good stretch, roll onto your right side and sit up slowly. Take your time. Place the petalite on a sunny windowsill or in moonlight to cleanse it.

TANZANITE: Altered states of consciousness

Tanzanite is a beautiful blue-violet gemstone and was first discovered in Tanzania, in East Africa. It balances the energies of the mind and the heart. It is often very expensive but small, rough or polished tumble stones can be found at gem suppliers. Some crystal healers declare it to be the most valuable crystal for metaphysics.

Use in Healing:
It activates and balances all the chakras, including those above the crown chakra, in the etheric body. It makes a good gemstone essence for meditation and healing. It stimulates

Meditation with Tanzanite

An earth healing meditation for the planet, using tanzanite. This meditation was given to me by the Angel of Earth Healing after the tsunami and earthquake in south-east Asia in 2004 and was used in many groups at the time.

Lie in relaxation and place a tanzanite gemstone over the heart chakra or the third eye. Tune in to your breathing. Notice each breath as it comes and goes. Then direct each breath into the gemstone. As you attune more and more to the tanzanite, you see a path of silvery light appear in front of you. You start to follow the path as it spirals higher and higher. You come to a splendid gateway. Visualize the wrought metalwork of gold and silver. Two angels guard the gate, one on each side.

You realize also that your own guardian angel is beside you, too. You are asked to give the password to open the gates. The password is DIVINE LOVE. You radiate divine love from your heart chakra, feeling it extend to all divine and sentient beings. The gates swing open and you go into a magnificent building.

It is formed of light and colour. The predominant colour is blue, but shot through with silver. You see a magnificent angelic being, with the Planet Earth at her heart centre and realize it is Gaia herself, the spiritual body of the planet. Use tanzanite to connect with this angel. Send love and healing to her. See the places that have been affected by recent earthquakes and wars being mended and healed. See the people of Planet Earth shaking hands and embracing each other in friendship and co-operation. As you do so, you notice that the planet is developing into a beautiful lotus blossom, the flower of enlightenment. The heart centre of Gaia is a beautiful lotus flower with the earth in its centre. She is healed by the divine love of her living people.

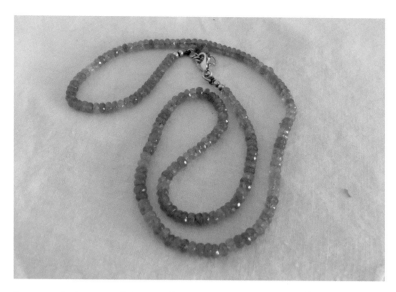

inner wisdom and is good to wear or carry to align the aura with higher states of consciousness. It combines well with iolite, danburite and moldavite to clear old karmic disease patterns and allows new patterns to integrate quickly.

Archangels and angels:
Tanzanite facilitates communication with higher beings of your choice.

Affirmation:

I now open to enlightened states of reality. This is released to me in perfect and harmonious ways, under grace and in divine right order.

Using the high-vibration crystals and working with angels can bring powerful healing and transformation to Planet Earth. Because crystals and gemstones are from the earth, they form a delightful companionship with the angels, a true bridge between heaven and earth.

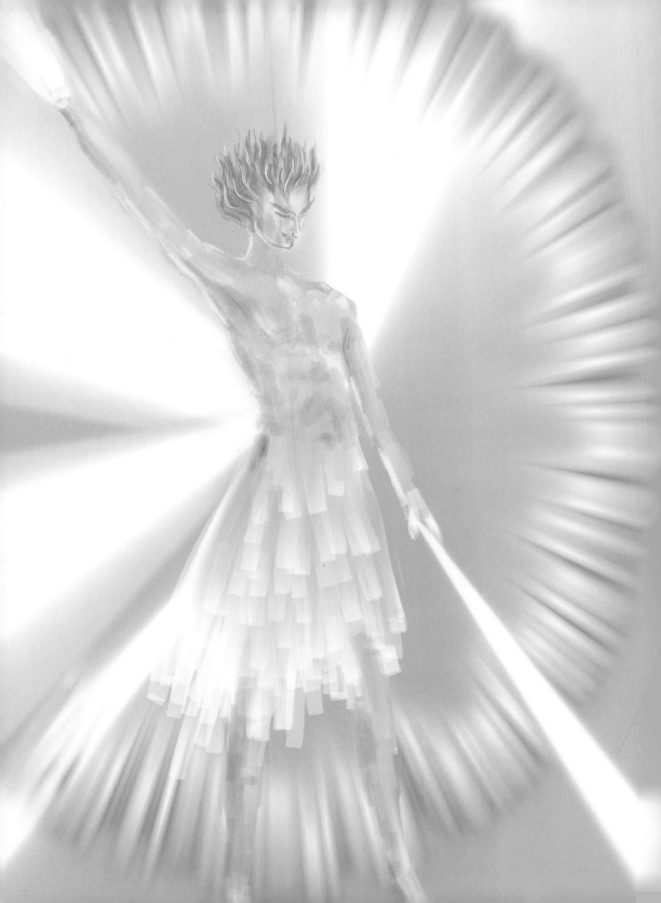

10.
Planetary Healing

We are the bridge from Spirit to Matter
You are the bridge from Matter to Spirit
You live in two worlds and we are your partners

JUST AS EACH of us has our own guardian or personal angel, there are national angels. As we saw, these are of the order known as principalities. Traditionally they are most concerned with Planet Earth, along with archangels and angels. Principalities are like guardian angels or caretakers of large groups of people, such as cities, counties, provinces, districts, towns, villages and even houses. They oversee the recent development of multinational companies. According to Pseudo-Dionysius, who lived long before the era of multinationals, they are also concerned with politics and religions. They help to inspire political leaders, both local and national, as well as the CEOs of multinational companies, to work for the good of humanity. In the world of religions, the principalities encourage prayer and meditation, seeking to inspire those who are devoted to God.

One of the great responsibilities of angels is bringing ideas and plans into physical form. At the highest level, this is co-creating with God, the Source of All-That Is, the universe itself, the galaxies, the stars and planets. At a human level, they are assisting us to bring our vision into physical life and practical expression. Like archangels and angels, they are most likely to have direct contact with people. Principalities are also likely to work through the archangels and angels.

Some of our great concerns at the moment are climate change, sustainability, pollution and other issues surrounding healthy living. At the same time that we are doing our best to think positively, and make changes in our lifestyle, we are surrounded by negative messages from the media and people around us. Many people are now trying to improve their lifestyle to conserve the resources of Planet Earth. Ancient spiritual traditions tell us that even two people working together for good can make changes, because God is with them.

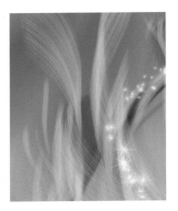

'I tell you that if two of you on earth agree about anything you ask for, it will be done for you by my Father in Heaven. For where two or three come together in my name, there am I with them.' Matthew 18 : 19–20

'We said once that the positive God-thought of one individual had greater power than the negative nebulous thought of ten thousand people. You have it in your own power to test the truth of our words. By your thought you can affect your own body and your own conditions and circumstances, and remould your life.'
White Eagle, in *Angelus* (magazine), July 1943

Groups of people working in co-operation are helping to save threatened species of animals and plants, the environment and the rainforest. Large charities have dramatically improved farm animal welfare in the countries where they operate. Such a movement is the charity, Compassion in World Farming, which campaigns for humanitarian treatment of farm animals and battery hens. It also campaigns against long journeys for farm animals, which cause animals and birds suffering and death. It began with one small farmer in 1967 and is now a global lobbying organization.

Local groups make changes for the better by setting up farmers' markets, renting allotments or collecting litter. People take over derelict land to clear it and plant vegetables—there is a major scheme for that in Detroit, in the USA, as I write. Environmental groups clear blocked rivers and streams and work to clean the water so fish return.

One person with vision, with ideas, who communicated

Brainstorm ten
ways in which
your local
community
is working
to improve
conditions.
(If you're not
sure, you can
look in the local
library, school or
college or check
the website
of your local
authority.)

Now brainstorm
ten things that
you already
do, or can do,
in your work,
home life or the
local community,
to improve or
preserve the
resources of the
area.

it to others, started each and every initiative. Perhaps the vision came to them from their personal team of angels and is even part of the plan they made before incarnating on earth. Before we are born, we decide what we will do. The act of birth then causes us to forget what we planned and we spend much of our lives remembering the plan. Having a spiritual awakening, or some kind of life crisis, is often part of the remembering process. Daily meditation and communing with angels helps us to remain in tune with what we came to do. Ancient traditions use rites of passage like the vision quest, when young people take some time alone to meditate and decide how they are to spend their lives.

In spite of people's best efforts, there are times of national or international difficulty. At such times, we can attune to the principalities for help.

When we attune, remarkable things sometimes come to us, as the experiences overleaf show. Yet it is not necessary to wait for emergencies to call on the principalities. We can use a regular meditation or prayer time to co-operate with them to help to heal the planet. Some meditation, prayer or healing groups meet regularly once a week or once a month to do this. There is an extra power in working together with like-minded people and angels to send healing and strength to continents, nations or cities. Even if you aren't part of a group, you will not be working alone, as the angels will be there with you. Remember to invite them. You can use the ideas that follow the two stories to start you off as a planetary healer.

When doing the directed meditation on pp. 164–5, if there are any countries or places that you feel need special help at any time, include them in your visualization and see the angel of that country or place beaming healing light and energy to it. Always try to work through the heart centre and leave the everyday worrying mind behind.

This is something that we can all do, either alone or with others, to help the earth and all the difficulties that can arise from time to time.

2001 Vision of Planetary Peace

As spiritual peacemakers, we need to keep the vision of peace alive, as we create the future with our positive thoughts and affirmations. Even when we hear about acts of violence, we can still continue with our meditations and affirmations and with visualizing peace. We can still visualize the picture of a peaceful planet and working in partnership with the angels. When enough of us do this, then it will come into reality. We create the vision and the path for others to follow. We don't need to be caught up in the drama of the media. Yes, we need to be informed, but we don't need to watch/listen/read about war or tragedies every hour.

In 2001, I was concerned after the tragedy of the bombing of the Twin Towers, the World Trade Centre, in New York. I sat in my study listening to a CD of music called 'Wolf Sister', by Marina Raye, a Native American flute player. As I listened, I left my body and had one of the most profound spiritual experiences I have ever had. It was completely spontaneous and lasted for an hour, although I was totally unaware of time passing. After it, I felt very uplifted. The feeling of spiritual encouragement from that experience is still with me nearly ten years later as I write. Here is what happened.

Listening to the music, I became aware that I was floating above Planet Earth. I could see her revolving, like a beautiful blue jewel, lit by the sun. No violence or terror was visible, only her radiant beauty. I could see far out into space and was aware of other planets, stars and galaxies. Then I could see four lines of white wolves approaching earth from the far distance of the universe. There was a line in each of the four directions— east, south, west and north. The lines of wolves seemed endless. As they reached the earth, they began to make a circle of protection. Soon there were four circles of wolves, circling in opposite directions around earth. I knew that the wolves symbolized protection. All wolves will always protect all the young of their pack. These white (spiritual) wolves are the protectors of earth and of us, first and foremost.

Then I saw four lines of young Native American warriors. They also marched towards earth and joined the wolves in their circle dance around the planet, so there were eight circles moving in opposite directions. The warriors are also protecting earth.

Four lines of wise men and four lines of wise women, healers and shamans, protectors of Planet Earth, followed the warriors. They represented all the races, cultures and traditions and all the ancient wisdom of earth. They reached the circles of wolves and warriors and joined them. In all, there were sixteen circles of dancers, moving in opposite directions.

Finally, I saw four lines of angels, moving towards earth from the four directions as before. They joined the circling dancers, in a wide-moving circle of protection around earth, so that there were now twenty circles of dancers travelling in opposite directions. Planet Earth, Gaia, is a virtue, one of the choirs of angels. To summarize this vision, it demonstrated to me that all the forces of light in the universe are always with us.

Star Vision

A few years ago, there was a terrorist bombing in London, the city where I live. On July 7th, 2005, I was in London for a meeting on the South Bank. The meeting never took place, as this was the day of the London bombings, now known as 7/7. I got to Waterloo Station and although Roy, my husband, tried to phone me to tell me there was no Underground train service, I didn't get the message. Having arrived at Waterloo about 10.00 a.m., there were announcements that people should not travel into London, but no information was given as to why. The station was full of passengers and police and the sirens of ambulances, fire engines and police vehicles filled the air. For those not familiar with London, Waterloo Station is right by St Thomas's Hospital, one of the leading London hospitals, and I knew later that many injured people were taken there. There were some train services going out of London and I got back home safely, wondering what was happening, as my mobile phone wasn't getting any signal, so I couldn't use it.

When I got back home, Roy told me what he knew from the news bulletins and I looked on the internet for more news. There was an email from my friend who said she had asked the help of angels for London. Roy and I did a White Eagle Lodge prayer for sending out the light, known as the Prayer for Humanity. I wondered what else I could do, not being able to spend the whole day in prayer and meditation. Then I thought about the Starlink website, www.thestarlink.net. I remembered that during the Second World War, the White Eagle Lodge had posters made and placed in the Underground Stations where people sheltered at night from the Blitz. I was guided to put the Star symbol, from the Starlink site, onto my computer screen. I emailed all my friends and contacts in my own meditation groups and yoga classes about it, giving them the link. I asked them to use it at any time during the day when they weren't using the computer for other work.

I realized that now, with modern technology, we can display this spiritual symbol anywhere, at all hours, and its energy will radiate throughout the places where it is needed. I put it on my own computer and it was there all afternoon, for five or six hours, as I remember. The interesting thing was that the computer never went into sleep mode, with a dark screen, which it is set to do after every few minutes or so when not in use. Every time I went to check it, the Star was still on the screen, golden and three-dimensional.

One of the abilities of principalities is to have greater strength from God to do what we might term miracles or unusual happenings, or things that cannot be explained—like computer screens not going blank! Many people also emailed me to say how helpful they found the image of the star to help them overcome their feelings of helplessness and even fear.

At 3.00 p.m., I did the Prayer for Humanity again and sent out the light, especially tuning in to the city of London. With my inner vision, I saw an immense star shining across the whole city. The star was the heart centre of an enormous angel, radiating healing light to the city. I could see numerous archangels, angels and spirit guides using the many rays of light, like paths, to enter into the city to inspire and encourage the rescue services in their work. The spiritual teacher, White Eagle, has always said that the angels and spirit messengers need our help to come to earth to help. I could see clearly how they did this.

One interesting follow-up to this is that there was another bombing attempt exactly two weeks later, but the bombs didn't go off. Also, the people of London, who now represent many different cultures and backgrounds, worked together to help each other throughout this period and after. Londoners were saying that no one would ever make them afraid to travel around their own city.

The next morning, I was again in London on business. I had to go into Waterloo again, but as there was no Underground service because of the emergency, I had to walk up to Covent Garden from the station. I passed cafes, pubs and restaurants that had notices outside, offering free food and accommodation as long as needed to those people who couldn't get home because of transport difficulties.

We can always call on the principalities whenever there is a crisis. They are the guardians of cities. Using three-dimensional graphic images like the Starlink one on computers helps us to visualize better when we are shocked, as it can be hard to concentrate.

PLANETARY AND NATIONAL HEALING

Sit or stand quietly, either alone or with a group of friends. If there are enough people, sit or stand in a circle. Light a candle and have some fresh flowers or a plant in the centre. You might like to burn essential oils or incense. Frankincense or sandalwood are good choices. It may help your attunement if you play suitable religious or New Age healing music before you start.

Breathe slowly and easily. Don't force your breath. Just let it flow in and out.

An essential requirement is to take your attention into the heart chakra. It is easier to contact angels through love and devotion. It also makes your attunement easier if you leave the everyday thoughts of the 'head mind' behind. Once you have established an easy regular breathing rhythm, follow the breath into the centre of your chest, into the heart chakra (centre). Allow the out-breath to flow out easily by relaxing your chest. Keep your posture lifted and erect, but not rigid and stiff.

When the breath is flowing easily and you are aware of the heart centre, begin to visualize a beautiful pink rose there. At its centre is a flame, the flame of the divine, which everyone has in his or her heart centre. Some people think of it as the Holy Spirit. Yogis call it Atman, the spark of God.

Continue the breathing, and visualize the flame growing larger and larger until it surrounds you and the group.

Call in the angels, archangels and principalities. Someone in the group could speak the words aloud. Make up your own suitable words, as angels like you to work from the heart. Here is an example.

'I (we) thank the angels, archangels and all the healing angels of Planet Earth for being here now to help in our work of healing the planet.'

Pause while you become attuned to the angels. You might feel their energy, see them, hear them or sense them. If your group wants to strengthen the attunement, hold hands. A recognized handhold for such group work is to hold your left hand palm up. Your right hand palm down covers the left palm of your neighbour.

One member of the group can speak suitable words now for healing of the earth. Begin by visualizing the earth, as a beautiful spinning globe, like the pictures taken from space. Send healing to earth, to the land. Visualize its beauty, the health of the rainforests, the fertility of the land, of the trees. Visualize everything as healthy and lush. Ask the angels to take the love energy of your heart centre to heal the land.

Now visualize the waters of the planet—lakes, rivers, oceans and seas. See them cleansed of all rubbish and pollution. Once again they are healthy, full of healthy living creatures. Send your angels with your love energy to heal the waters of the planet.

Visualize clean, fresh air, free from any pollution. Ask the angels to send your heart's love energy to the air, cleaning away dirt and debris. See it fresh and pure and perfect for earth's living creatures, including people, to breathe.

Visualize the earth now at the centre of a beautiful lotus of light, all healed and pure. See it surrounded by angels and held in perfection.

To close your attunement, release your hands and hold them together over your heart. Thank the angels for their help. Feel yourself surrounded by the love of the angels who have worked with you.

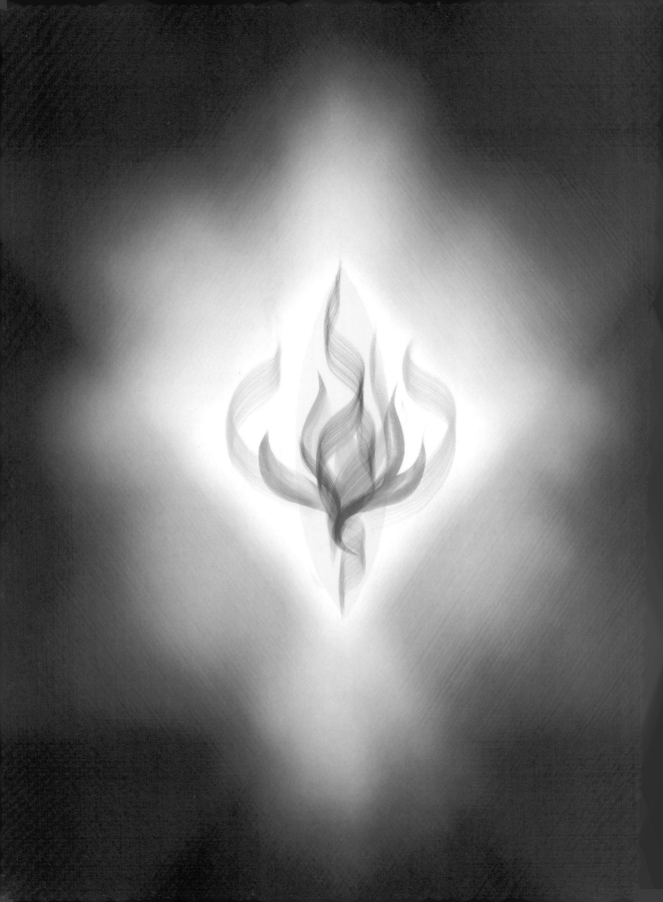

11.

The Golden Age

MYTHS and legends from all parts of the world refer to a past golden age when life was peaceful and harmonious. Angels and people worked in partnership together. The human race was seen as pure and lived in a state of peace and harmony, stability, prosperity and happiness. There was no sickness or disease. Goodness ruled, for there were no evil thoughts or bad behaviour. The yogis refer to this golden age as *satya yug* or *satya yuga*.

A golden age is seen as a time of heaven on earth, a Garden of Eden, or Utopia. In the case of the Eden we remember in myth, a time came when the human race needed to learn to be independent, so people learned to develop their own abilities. Life on earth became more testing in order that people would develop strength of character. History, as we know it, began.

Deep in their individual consciousness, people still long for that golden age, and when the partnership between people and angels is re-established, once again there will indeed be a golden age on earth. The way to bring it into being is—by working with the angels—to banish all discord and intolerance and to use the ability of creative imagination to picture it and so draw it close to us.

At the present time, we are living at the end of an age, which the yogis call *kali yuga*, the Age of Iron. The Mayans call it the time of no time. Have you ever wondered why so many people talk about having no time? The present years are also called the End Times, because of the end of the Mayan Calendar, and some people delight in discussing destructive prophecies. It is easy to be pulled into negative and destructive thoughts and ideas by what we see and hear. We can keep our own power by being independent and not allowing ourselves to be drawn into any of this negativity.

In 1987, there began astrologically a period of twenty-five years following an event that came to be called 'the Harmonic Convergence'. On August 17th, 1987, people all over the world meditated on earth healing and this unified energy of intention caused a new spiritual era to dawn. This event is said to have changed the history of the earth for ever. Ancient prophecies of the Hopi, Lakota Sioux and other Native Americans, as well as the Maya, foretold a time of twenty-five years, beginning on August 15th–17th, 1987, and leading up to 2012, when a spiritual initiation would enable humanity to expand their consciousness into a time of spiritual transformation. This twenty-five-year period seems to be a time of unparalleled spiritual interest. Books about spirituality, angels, spirit guides and self-help abound on the shelves of bookshops and libraries. Renewed interest in a change of consciousness to a more spiritual outlook can be seen in the interest on the Internet and in films. More centres and courses about meditation and spirituality open regularly. People discuss topics like meditation and angels more openly.

The Angel of the Golden Age

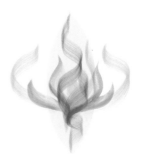

The Angel of the Golden Age is one of the order of angels known as virtues. This order is able to radiate divine power and energy to the human family to inspire them to work towards the right personal qualities needed at this time. It is often said that we can't change the world before we change ourselves.

Be the change you want to see!

The golden age angel also aids the work of lifting the vibrations of Planet Earth. Archangel Uriel also has particular responsibility for the planet and the environment and is known as the Angel of Gold.

This angel also aids the work of lifting the vibrations of Planet Earth. Archangel Uriel also has particular responsibility for the planet and the environment and is known as the Angel of Gold. One of his tasks is as the Angel of Salvation, not only of individuals, but also Planet Earth.

The Angel of the Golden Age holds the vision or blueprint of the age and all that it implies. It imparts the vision to those who can share it and begin to work towards it. The angel's message is this:

Begin to change yourself for the better. Continue with your spiritual and personal development and be certain that whatever you are doing is right for you. Introduce simple changes that you can make easily. Choose things that you are confident and comfortable about doing.

Eat pure, wholesome foods and drink fresh, pure water to cleanse your body. Begin to clear untidiness and clutter. Do it in small ways, perhaps beginning with the drawer that you have been meaning to tidy. Do it bit by bit. Give generously to charity shops of the things you no longer need so others with less means can enjoy them. Surround yourself with simple and beautiful things and keep your home clean and tidy; introduce beautiful plants and calming, relaxing music to keep your home restful and pure, so that you enjoy being in it and people will be happy to be with you.

Meditate and attune to the angelic kingdom and the world of the golden age to become familiar with its ideals and goals. Use affirmations to make the building blocks that create the golden age. Remember the power of your thoughts, your imagination.

You are co-creators with the Source of All-That-Is. Whatever you think, will be. If you think depressing, miserable thoughts and play fearful scenes in your mind, fear and depression are what you create in your life. Use the law of attraction to draw into your life the things you need. Write or draw your plans in a notebook and read it and work in it often, daily if possible.

If you continually aim to have happy thoughts, to use positive affirmations and practise kindness and love towards others, then the golden age will begin in your own life and spread to those around you. Thought by thought, day by day, the world can be changed for the better and the golden age will be ushered in.

When you catch yourself having aggressive thoughts towards those who upset you, change your thoughts until you no longer feel the aggression. Surround yourself with pure golden white light and send it to them. An easy way to do this is to bless the person by saying, 'Bless you, bless you, and bless you'. Do this constantly, until it becomes second nature to surround yourself and others with light. Then notice how your moods lift and better things start to appear in your life.

Create a corner in a room where you can meditate and tune in easily to the spirit worlds and the angels. Light a candle, burn incense or pure essential oils in a vaporizer. Place a beautiful crystal, flowers or plants there. Use this special place every day, even if it's only for five minutes. Then the angelic energy builds and the angels can use it to come nearer to you to inspire you with their ideas. Angels will come close to you and work with you and give you the keys that you can use.

The angels and archangels will be delighted when we collaborate with them and work towards the golden age, so that once again we live in a world of beauty, harmony and peace. They will help us to usher in the divine qualities of freedom and liberty, justice and equality. These are divine gifts that help people to overcome fears of suffering, so that people will learn to work together in harmony to develop responsibilities as well as human rights.

Opposite, to close, are some words from the Angel of the Golden Age.

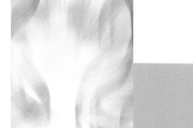

A Golden Age Angel Message

Call me Aurelia.
See my golden aura,
My colours
That radiate forth.
I am like the rising sun
For my aura radiates
Its golden liquid rays
And enfold you and all humanity.
These rays of golden light
Fill you as they enter your lungs and heart
On your breath.
Visualize the golden colour of this subtle energy
And feel the beneficial effect
Of this energy in your system.
As I overshadow you
My rays of gold fill you like the sun
When it rises in the morning
And chases away the dark shadows.
My rays of loving, golden light
Dissolve old hurts and sorrows,
The shadows that have accumulated in your being.
And like the sun,
Your aura radiates beautiful shades of gold
For you are the sun of your universe
And the golden age of your life
Takes birth in you.

Meditation with the Angel of the Golden Age

A BAPTISM OF GOLDEN LIGHT

Prepare your meditation space with a gold candle and yellow flowers, music, incense or essential oils and sit quietly, centring yourself with smooth, gentle breathing.

Visualize a brilliant light, like the sun, above your head. As you breathe, draw it down until it surrounds you and fills you with radiant light. See light filling every cell of your whole being, until you find yourself radiating light from each cell, like millions of tiny suns.

In front of you now is a path of light. Walk along the path. You move effortlessly, as if on a moving pavement. In the distance is an even more brilliant golden light, coming closer as you move towards it. It is one of the angels working with the Angel of the Golden Age. It has come to take you to a ceremony of gold.

It is like the sun, ablaze with golden light. Light pours from its aura and heart. Its eyes are filled with love and also radiate light. You see many different shades of gold, yellow and white, the very highest spiritual colours. This golden light is like an essence that revitalizes you, renews your energy and cleanses your bloodstream, washing away all tiredness and stress from your physical body.

As you go with the angel it is as if you are entering the sun itself, so brilliant is the light, yet it doesn't dazzle you. You see before you a magnificent building, like a university or cathedral. Take some time to examine it and see its architectural designs and qualities. It is unlike anything you have ever seen before.

You go into the building with the angel guide and into a large auditorium. Many people are waiting on seats, all accompanied by an angel guide. All around the walls are flowers, like lilies and roses in different shades of gold and white. The air is filled with their sweet perfume. Subtle sounds of music seem to playing in the background.

Now a magnificent being appears at the front of the auditorium: the Angel of the Golden Age. This angel is so large, it seems to be as tall as the building itself. It radiates a special light from its golden heart centre. The light bathes you and enters into every part of your being, dissolving away all the weariness, depression, guilt and negativity that you have ever felt. Identify any negative feelings or memories that you particularly wish to release. Visualize the golden essence of light dissolving it away, filling you with light. Breathe in the golden light, filling your bloodstream and every cell with it. You feel renewed and uplifted.

The angel now asks if you are willing to work to bring in the golden age. You will be asked to do only what is easy for you. Take some time to reflect on this and tell the angel what you plan to do. Choose something that is easy to achieve, for you can always improve on it later. You can come here any time you like for healing and inspiration.

It is time to go now. As you look down at yourself, you realize that you are wearing a beautiful golden robe of light. Your body of light, your aura, has become more enlightened. The angel guide leads you out of the building and along the moving pathway of light until you are once again aware of your meditation place.

Close down in your usual way, have a drink of water to ground yourself, and take time to return to your everyday duties.

12.
Epilogue

ROY WAS scheduled for major abdominal surgery in the local hospital. The doctors were also worried about his slow heart rate and so he went to the cardiology department early in the morning before the operation. He had an angiogram and a temporary pacemaker. Then he went to the operating theatre. Eventually I managed to get news about him and was given permission to visit him in the Intensive Care Unit in the evening.

A nursing sister came to see me. She explained that Roy was bleeding very badly and would have to go back to the operating theatre for another operation to find where the bleeding was. She said I could see him for a few minutes. I was very shocked when I saw him. There was a lot of blood and he was shaking violently. He had an oxygen mask and drips and all the other paraphernalia that an ICU has to use. Machines that beeped constantly surrounded him. I held his hand and he kept squeezing it. Then the doctor asked me to leave so they could operate. They asked me what his religion was, which really alarmed me. It was on all his paperwork anyway, but I thought it meant he would need a minister urgently.

I went home and sent out emails and messages on my Facebook page for urgent healing for Roy. Nearly all our friends and contacts are healers, meditators, yoga practitioners and believers of various faiths. With the internet we could send one message to all our contacts at the same time—such a time saver. Before I went to bed I had a lot of messages of support and more the next morning. A continual chain of prayer and healing was set up for him.

I only slept for about two hours and then woke up. I was freezing cold, and although it was August I had to put on winter pyjamas and socks. People who know me well know that I don't feel the cold, so it was unusual for me to react like

HAND IN HAND WITH ANGELS

this. My heart was pounding in my chest and I could hear it in my ears. My whole body seemed to be throbbing. I made some hot chocolate but still couldn't get warm. I lay in bed with the duvet wrapped tightly around me.

Then I was in the tunnel of light with Roy. It was filled with angels. The light was very bright but it didn't dazzle. We were moving through the light until we came to a beautiful garden, but the angels wouldn't let me in. It was a beautiful garden, but it wasn't my time to go in. I had to leave Roy there and come back along the tunnel. I was sobbing violently but I knew that if it was his time to return home to the light, I had to let him go. I told the angels I wouldn't hold him back if he had to go on. Roy had to make the decision himself whether he would go or stay and I had to come back along the tunnel. I told him I would manage and he mustn't worry about me. I was still shivering and cold. I was aware of angels with me all the time. I seemed to be between the two worlds. Then again, I was in the tunnel of light with Roy. The same thing happened. I had to leave him at the entrance to the garden and return. I did not sleep again that night. I found out later that several of my friends who are healers were also awake at the same time and thinking of Roy. One of them emailed me after hearing my story, thanking me, as she thought it was only her imagination, but now knew it was a real experience.

This happened as I was doing the proofs for this book, so I was in the position of having to read and put into practice all that I teach in a time of crisis. Two important things stand out from this. I want to call the tunnel 'the tunnel of Love'. I think that's what it is, because we all return to the perfect love from which we were created. The other thing is that we never need to be afraid of our human vulnerability at these times of crisis. Call on all your angels and spiritual guides for help. Even if you are too emotional to see them or be aware of them, they are always with you. You only need to ask. We are never alone.

A week later, Roy is slowly recovering. Even as I write, he only knows that the doctors told him it was 'touch and go' with him on that night. He doesn't remember anything or that I was with him in the ICU.

INDEX